Ovarian Cancer Journeys

❖

Survivors Share Their Stories
To Help Others

Edited by
Ayala Miron

iUniverse, Inc.
New York Lincoln Shanghai

Ovarian Cancer Journeys
Survivors Share Their Stories To Help Others

iUniverse, Inc.

For information address:
iUniverse, Inc.
2021 Pine Lake Road, Suite 100
Lincoln, NE 68512
www.iuniverse.com

ISBN: 0-595-33031-2

Printed in the United States of America

This book is dedicated:

To the survivors having the courage to revisit and share their true stories on their ovarian cancer journeys.

To my husband Ami who is standing by me, I am so blessed to have your love and support.

To my children Benjamin, Jonathan, Michelle, and David, you help make my life meaningful everyday.

Contents

AKNOWLEGEMENTS

Thanks to the women survivors who took their time to write the details of their ovarian cancer journeys. We met and shared our experiences, from symptoms, to diagnosis, trough treatment, and survival. Their contributions made this book possible.

Thanks to Betty Reiser and Robin Cohen for introducing me to some of the survivors.

Thanks to Barbara A. Goff, MD, for writing the introduction and for leading research on ovarian cancer symptoms, and to Ann Schlagenhauf for her assistance.

Thanks to Amy Levine, MD, Rachel Zuckerman, Melissa Dobbyn, Meg Gains, and Elizabeth Shamir, for reviewing and giving feedback and comments on the manuscript of this book.

Thanks to the dedicated and knowledgeable medical professionals from whom I have learned about ovarian cancer: Jhon Kavanagh MD, Ralph S. Freedman MD, Benjamin Lichtiger MD, Parviz Hanjani MD, Susan Nolte RN-PhD, Robert Ozols MD, Stephen C. Rubin MD, Ross Berkowitz MD, Lois Almadrones RN, Richard Barakat MD, Julie Esch RN, Katherine O Flaherty RN, and Paul Sabbatini MD.

Thanks to Ami Miron who encouraged and supported me during this project. Thanks to Benjamin Miron for doing the web site design of this book with Michelle Miron—www.ocjourneys.com. Thanks to Jonathan Miron for creating the design of the front and back covers. Thanks to David Miron for being proud of this book.

Ayala Miron

FOREWORD

✦

Ayala Miron

Many of us try to stay healthy by following the advice of health care professionals. We do our best to eat well, exercise regularly, avoid stress, and go for regular medical checkups. Most of us believe that these measures will contribute to better health, but they are no guarantees against cancer.

I was diagnosed with advanced ovarian cancer, In April 2000, when I was 43 years old. I had been living a healthy lifestyle and had followed the advice of my health care providers. During the last few years before my diagnosis, I had complained of recurring physical symptoms to my doctors, which I describe later in this book. They assured me repeatedly that I was in great shape, and could find nothing wrong with me. All throughout that time, my doctors dutifully recorded in great detail the symptoms I had. They did not suggest other evaluation tests, until I had to go to the emergency room.

As it turned out, my health care providers had repeatedly misdiagnosed my symptoms. They didn't know enough about ovarian cancer and did not suspect that my complaints were serious. After my ovarian cancer diagnosis, I realized that this disease caused the symptoms I felt. I also learned that many health care providers mistakenly consider ovarian cancer "a silent disease." My symptoms, over a number of years, taught me differently.

Since my diagnosis, I have met many ovarian cancer experts in the medical community who have helped me to learn more about this disease. As I met ovarian cancer survivors, I realized that we had common ideas and insight on how ovarian cancer can be detected early. We joined in this book to share our stories and to help others understand better this disease.

Ovarian cancer specialists agree that early detection is critical for long-term survival. Unfortunately, the statistics tell another story. In the United States 75% of women with ovarian cancer are diagnosed with a late stage disease, when their cancer has spread beyond the ovaries. Ovarian cancer is the deadliest of all gynecologic cancers and the fourth leading cause of cancer death among US women[1].

We can change that. Ovarian cancer is highly curable when detected early. Currently there is no easy way to detect ovarian cancer because there is no screening test for this disease. The CA-125 blood test, used to help detect ovarian cancer, is not reliable enough. More research is needed to develop a better screening test for early detection. Recent independent scientific studies results show that 89% of women with ovarian cancer, experienced symptoms at the early stages of the disease. This means that symptoms occur in the early stages of the disease when this cancer can be cured. Ovarian cancer symptoms can no longer be ignored. Being aware of and listening to the warning signs and symptoms of ovarian cancer, can lead to many more cases of early detection and cure.

Most women with ovarian cancer, over 90% of all cases, do not have any close relative with the disease, they don't know much about it, and are caught by surprise when they find out that they have ovarian cancer. Therefore, it is important for women to learn about the warning signs and symptoms of ovarian cancer, and to be persistent in pursuing proper diagnostic tests and medical care, immediately when they feel something is wrong. They need to trust their bodies, and to act as their own advocates with their health care providers.

Health care providers too, need to heed the complaints of their patients. Many of the survivors in this book volunteer in medical school nationwide, where we share our stories with third-year medical students, to bring about a better understanding and awareness of this disease. Our stories illustrate ovarian cancer can be detected early when health care providers know enough about the disease, listen to their patients complaints of symptoms, perform thorough physical exams, and use appropriate diagnostic tools.

The stories in this book are visceral, strong, and above all, true. Our intention is to help others by sharing our experiences. We hope that patients, their relatives, healthy women, and members of the medical community will have a deeper insight into this disease after reading our stories and considering lessons we have learned. Ultimately, we hope to help bring about a better future, starting with early detection, for those diagnosed with ovarian cancer.

Ayala Miron
September 1, 2004

---

1. American Cancer Society, Cancer Statistics—2004.
    See resources for more information.

INTRODUCTION

✦

Barbara A. Goff, MD

It is an honor to be asked to contribute to this important collection of stories. As a gynecologic oncologist, I have dedicated myself to the research and treatment of gynecologic malignancies. Six years ago through a chance encounter with an inspirational ovarian cancer survivor, I became interested in studying symptoms and early diagnosis of ovarian cancer.

In 1998 I met Cindy Melancon, editor of *Conversations Newsletter* for those fighting ovarian cancer. During an educational conference for the lay public, Cindy and other survivors challenged the notion that ovarian cancer was a silent disease. After listening to these survivors' exceptional stories, I decided to team up with Cindy so that we could evaluate symptoms and early diagnosis in a scientific manner. During medical school, residency and even gynecologic oncology fellowship I had been taught that ovarian cancer was a silent disease and so initially I was not optimistic that our studies would yield new information.

The results of our first study were published in the *Journal of Cancer* in November of 2000. Is this study over 1725 women with ovarian cancer were surveyed about their symptoms and how the disease was diagnosed. In response to the question whether or not patients had symptoms before the diagnosis of ovarian cancer, only 5% of patients reported they had none, 61% reported increased abdominal size, 57% abdominal bloating, 47% fatigue, 36% abdominal pain, 31% indigestion, 27% urinary frequency, 26% pelvic pain, 25% constipation, 24% urinary incontinence, 23% back pain, 17% pain with intercourse, 16% unable to eat normally, 14% vaginal bleeding, 11% weight loss, and 9% nausea. When we evaluated the response of symptoms by stage of disease, we found that 89% of those in Stage I did report symptoms; and for Stage III and IV, the rate was 97%. This finding was significant because women with early stage ovarian cancer are not supposed to have symptoms, according to most major textbooks. The other reason that this is significant is that women with early stage disease (Stage I and Stage II) have a cure rate of 70-90%. In contrast, women with advanced stage disease (Stage III and Stage IV) have a cure rate of only 20-30%, so the early identification of ovarian cancer based on symptoms could significantly improve survival.

Other results from our survey revealed that, unfortunately, even when women brought their abnormal symptoms to the attention of their physician, many were initially misdiagnosed as having other conditions. Thirteen percent of survey participants were told by their physician that their symptoms really were not related to anything at all; 15% were told they had irritable bowel; 12% were told that they were stressed out; 6% were diagnosed with depression; and another 15% were diagnosed with other gastrointestinal disorders. A full 30% of women were treated for other conditions prior to their diagnosis, and 64% indicated that there were barriers. When patients were asked to elaborate, 22% responded that they personally ignored their symptoms; 30% reported that the wrong diagnosis was made; 21% reported health care provider's attitude towards them was a problem; and 6% reported difficulty getting an appointment. Physicians were able to make a diagnosis of ovarian cancer in 0-2 months in 55% of cases; in 19% of patients it took 3-6; in 15% of patients it took 7-12 months; and, in 11% of patients it took greater than 12 months to make the diagnosis. As time to make the diagnosis increased, the percentage of women who were diagnosed with advanced stage disease significantly increased as well.

The importance of this study was that it showed definitely that women with ovarian cancer, even with early stage disease, do have symptoms. This is in direct contrast to what is stated in most textbooks and taught in most medical schools. The symptoms most commonly seen are those related to abdominal and gastrointestinal complaints, and not necessarily "gynecologic" in nature. Many women stated that they attributed their symptoms to menopause, getting older, or the stress of multiple demands on their lives. Women are often unaware of what constitutes normal physiologic changes with aging as opposed to pathologic changes. Clearly, this is an area where public education efforts need to focus. Sadly, health care provider delay can also be a problem. The lack of information that ovarian cancer can cause symptoms, and the vague symptoms that ovarian cancer patients often present with, can mislead health care providers. As a result, patients get treated for other non-specific diseases, and so educational efforts also need to target health care providers. This study also suggests that we may be best able to reduce delays in diagnosis by better educating both patients and health care providers about the symptoms of ovarian cancer.

Following the publication of our study, investigators at Memorial Sloan Kettering published a case control study evaluating symptoms in women with ovarian cancer. Their study confirmed our initial findings and importantly, they also found that 89% of women with early stage disease had symptoms.

Recently (June 2004), we published in JAMA another study evaluating symptoms of ovarian cancer in women who present to primary care clinics and compared them to women with ovarian cancer who were surveyed prior to surgery. In this study we found that symptoms of ovarian cancer are commonly found in women who present to primary care clinics, which may be one reason physicians have such a difficult time making a diagnosis of ovarian cancer. However, women with ovarian cancer were significantly more likely to have symptoms that were more severe, more frequent and of more recent onset than women in the clinic population. In addition, cancer patients were more likely to have co-existence of symptoms, particularly bloating, increased abdominal size and urinary symptoms. With this research we are beginning to quantify the differences in symptoms that women with ovarian cancer experience. We hope in future studies to develop an ovarian cancer symptom index that could be used by primary care providers to help identify symptom patterns that need prompt evaluation.

All of the research has reinforced that ovarian cancer is not a silent disease as was once thought and as is shown quite eloquently in this collection of stories. However, we need to do more to educate both women and providers about the early warning signs. We also need to push for more research support so that investigators can continue to work on prevention, early diagnosis and treatment of this devastating disease.

The value of this collection of stories is that it helps raise awareness about symptoms, need for patient persistence, and the importance of being treated by a gynecologic oncologist. As this collection shows, it is important for women to advocate for themselves and it is essential for women with suspected ovarian cancer to receive care from physicians with specialized training in gynecologic cancers (gynecologic oncologists). Numerous studies have shown a significant survival advantage for women with ovarian cancer who receive their cancer surgery from these specialists. The Gynecologic Cancer Foundation (www.wcn.org) is a non-profit organization that is dedicated to educating women about ovarian cancer and other gynecologic malignancies. It is a wonderful resource that provides information regarding risk factors, diagnosis, treatment, and how to locate specialists in your area. Until we find ways to prevent ovarian cancer, early detection and treatment by appropriate physician specialists will give women the best chance of fighting this disease.

Barbara A. Goff, MD

Professor and Co-Director, Division of Gynecologic Oncology
University of Washington School of Medicine, Seattle, WA

IMPORTANCE OF A SPECIALIST

❖

Karen

Diagnosed at age 49
In May 2001
With epithelial ovarian cancer
Stage IIIC

In 2001, I had been an intensive care nurse for the previous 28 years, yet, like most women, I knew virtually nothing about ovarian cancer. I did know it is one of the deadliest forms of cancers, from watching a character named Nancy battling this disease in the old TV show "Thirtysomething," and the fact that Gilda Radner had died from it. I was pretty punctual with my annual gynecological exams. When I was in my late 30s, I was diagnosed with fibroids. They were not unusual, since fibroids ran in my family. Over the next 10 years, I had two ultrasounds done to check on their progress, the last ultrasound was performed in 1998.

In March 2000, I went for my annual exam. That fall, I began having periods that lasted 10 days and bad menstrual cramps. I had never suffered from bad menstrual cramps before, but the acute abdominal pains I started to feel, could literally stop me in my tracks. I remember being in such terrible pain one day at work in the ICU (Intensive Care Unit), that I called my gynecologist from there. He phoned in a prescription for a painkiller called Anaprox, which did not help at all. However, I chose to persevere with the pain. After all, I was 48, and I thought that menopause had to be the reason for these symptoms.

In March 2001, I returned to my gynecologist for my annual exam. As soon as he palpated my abdomen, his initial remark was that the fibroids had grown quite a bit.

I was scheduled for an ultrasound on Thursday, April 12, 2001. I remember lying on the table in the ultrasound room. The tech doing the test told me that he would show me the huge masses on my ovaries, because as a nurse, he thought I would not panic. At that moment, my life changed forever as I fought to keep panic at bay. I knew then that it was cancer. That evening my doctor called saying he wanted to see me in the office the next day to schedule surgery and take some additional tests.

My husband accompanied me to the office the following morning. A CBC (Complete Blood Count) blood test, which showed me to be anemic, and a CA-125 blood test, which would be in the 900s, were drawn. My gynecologist also wanted me to choose one of the general surgeons from the small community hospital where we both worked, in case he discovered that my colon or small intestines were involved. I complied and chose the general surgeon.

I remember going home that afternoon and feeling almost passive due to the shock of it all.

My three sisters, unbeknown to me, had been gathering info and rallying behind my back. There was no way my possible cancer surgery was going to be done at a community hospital by an obstetrician gynecologist, if they could help it.

They immediately called two well-known cancer centers, searching for a gynecologic oncologist surgeon. One of them told me to fax my ultrasound to them immediately, which I did. An appointment was obtained in a flash.

Further lab work was performed, which revealed my platelets were around the one million mark, which is considered dangerously high and risky for surgery. A hematology oncologist was called on, and another primary cancer source was sought. After further labs and a bone marrow biopsy, the doctor determined that an active disease in my pelvis caused my thrombocytosis (high level of thrombocytes or platelets in the blood, causing blood cloths to form). I went on Agrylin to lower the platelets.

From the time of the ultrasound to my surgery date, I waited seven weeks. My actual debulking surgery took around six hours. My cancer involved both ovaries and one lymph node. All other pathologies were normal. My gynecology oncologist informed me that if my surgery had been done at the community hospital, the infected lymph node would likely have been missed, and I would have been diagnosed with a much earlier stage of cancer and been deathly ill within a year. Instead, after the surgery, I had no sign of visible disease.

In hindsight and after educating myself extensively on ovarian cancer, I realized I had quite a few of the symptoms commonly found in ovarian cancer patients. Among them were lower backaches (which I mistakenly attributed to my long hours as a nurse), weird pains in my thighs, frequent urination, as well as the symptoms that I attributed to oncoming menopause.

But what hurt me the most, was that my gynecologist, who worked with me in the same hospital, and with whom I had an ongoing relationship, would have taken my life literally in his hands to perform this surgery on me. Clearly, the indicators were quite strong for ovarian cancer. Did he not know that by performing the surgery he could have greatly reduced my odds for survival? During that first phone conversation we had, after the ultrasound, he should have immediately sent me to a gynecologic oncologist surgeon.

I completed chemotherapy in October 2001. I am fortunate that today in 2004, I am still showing no signs of the disease. I realize that my future remains uncertain. I live each three-month interval between checkups to the fullest.

I want to do my part to make sure that every woman knows the symptoms of ovarian cancer, and the importance of gynecologic oncologists.

The advice I received from my oncologist *for women at risk of ovarian cancer* to protect themselves from this disease is to be followed by their doctor with: vaginal ultrasounds, CA-125 blood tests (unless a better screening test becomes available), and complete pelvic recto/vaginal exams. To reduce the chances of ovarian cancer he also suggested for some women to take birth control pills, for five years *might help.*

OVARIAN CANCER SYMPTOMS

✦

Marsha

Diagnosed at age 45
In August 1995
With ovarian cancer
Stage IV

As a nine-year survivor of Stage IV ovarian cancer, I am happy to be here—in 2004—and in fact, I am happy to be anywhere.

Ovarian cancer can be curable, especially if caught at an early enough stage. But in most cases, because there is no reliable, routine screening test and because there is a long-standing notion that there are no early symptoms, it is often relegated to being a last-resort diagnosis. It is difficult to diagnose this disease early because its symptoms are very commonplace for women and are often either minimized or dismissed. All of the symptoms women with ovarian cancer experience are very likely, especially on a difficult day, to sound almost whiny or emotion-driven.

Unfortunately, the symptoms of ovarian cancer: bloating, gas, constipation, indigestion, nausea, urinary frequency and urgency, abdominal cramping, leg and back pain, and fatigue often fall in the category of being a "nuisance" and not "life-threatening." They are so deceptively simple that both physicians and patients often feel comfortable explaining them away.

Urinary frequency was the primary symptom I had. I don't think people realize that it can be a symptom of ovarian cancer. An example of people making light of this symptom is how it's portrayed in a TV commercial for the medication Detrol, as being almost comical, with women unable to get to a bathroom as the "Gotta go, gotta go, gotta go" jingle plays in the background. In addition, gas and indigestion, two other symptoms of ovarian cancer, can be minimized with a myriad of prescription and over-the counter drugs.

Because the symptoms may affect more than one system, patients often go to an internist, gynecologist, and gastroenterologist, and this can compromise follow-up. Probably one of the most valuable instruments in diagnosing ovarian cancer are a physician's listening skills and knowledge of ovarian cancer symptoms, which can often be misconstrued as being something less serious. How many times have women experienced bloating or cramping since their first period? Physicians should ask patients who complain of these symptoms (and themselves) why these ailments felt different enough that day, to make them take time off from work to see a doctor.

Although that's not a whole lot for a physician to go on, the dual nature of these symptoms—that they are common, but are somehow different enough to make them seek medical attention—should be a red flag for ovarian cancer.

I hope that women and their physicians can learn about the symptoms of ovarian cancer better when they hear about them from survivors, and that it will help women and their doctors to be more aware of those symptoms.

The following are symptoms, women have experienced from one year to several months before ovarian cancer diagnosis. Some of them are quotes from the late comedian Gilda Radner's book "It's Always Something," some are from women in my support group, and the last quote is mine.

- I would wake up feeling as if I was getting the flu, only I would never come down with it. I would feel okay the next day, and then a week later, feel like I was getting something again.

- I experienced uncontrollable fatigue, sometimes, strong enough so that I could not get out of bed. My doctor said it was nerves, since I was recently divorced. My internist thought it was Epstein-Barr virus, although he said he did not really believe there was such a thing as this disease. He also thought my symptoms might be from depression. He told me to "Just relax, it'll burn itself out."

- Sometimes I would run a fever, which my doctor said can happen with Epstein-Barr virus.

- I felt weird all the time, even worse around my period.

- I had weird pelvic cramping. My gynecologist said it was mittelschmerz.

- I had pains in my stomach and bowel. My gynecologist said it was definitely a stomach problem, and referred me to a gastroenterologist who told me my gas was caused by taking Vitamin C. He also thought my problem was emotional, or related to food allergies.

- I had aching, gnawing pains in my upper thighs and legs. The gynecologist and gastroenterologist could find no reason for it. My blood tests were normal.

- Although I was on a diet, my clothes were getting tight around the waist. The doctor said my body was changing with age, and I was probably cheating on my diet.

- I had the urge to urinate constantly. The doctor said it was a symptom of menopause. I had such urinary frequency, I could not get a good night's sleep. The doctor said I had a "sensitive bladder."

In 1994, at the age of 45, I was treated for months with Pyridium to reduce my bladder sensitivity and was reassured that this was nothing serious, just a nuisance that would eventually go away. When I went back to the doctor six months later, she detected a pelvic mass. After I had a sonogram, I received a phone call from her telling me I had advanced ovarian cancer.

Of all the emotions that I experienced at that moment: shock, fear, disbelief, anger, the most overwhelming was the feeling of suddenly becoming cut off and separated from the rest of the world. Although physically I felt the same as I had before the phone rang, emotionally I felt as if now I was amongst the sick and possibly dying, and felt immobilized. I kept hearing her say "You have to have a CAT scan," and "You have to see an oncologist." Because she used the word "You" repeatedly, it validated a feeling that I alone had to take on this disease. She conveyed an urgency I felt unable to deal with. I know there is no easy way to break bad news to a patient, but if doctors said things like "*We* will schedule a CAT scan" or "*We* will get the appointment set up," it would convey support to their patients and help ease them into the terrifying whirlwind of activity that follows this devastating diagnosis.

Since that day in 1995, nine years ago, I have had three surgeries and two rounds of chemotherapy, one was for the original diagnosis and one for a recurrence three years later. Although I was diagnosed at Stage IV with a lymph node in my neck, I have had two complete responses to treatment and know that many women have not been as fortunate. Of all the ways that I am enjoying this period of my life, none is more gratifying than telling my story. I hope that telling people about my experiences and conveying the lessons I've learned from some remarkable women, will change the course of the disease for others.

THOROUGH MEDICAL CARE

✦

Barbara

Diagnosed at age 51
In August 1996
With ovarian cancer
Stage IC

I was diagnosed with ovarian cancer the way everyone should be—at stage one. During a routine physical exam my nurse practitioner did a rectal vaginal exam and discovered that I had an ovarian cyst. This raised a red flag in her mind that it might be ovarian cancer. I had not noticed any symptoms, beforehand. I went for a transvaginal ultrasound, and my gynecologist ordered a CA-125 blood test. She said to me "we are going to rule everything out" and her actions saved my life.

Six weeks later the cysts were gone, but because the CA-125 was still elevated, they began to monitor those levels. When my own doctor was away, her covering partner called with results from one of the CA-125 tests and said, "See, this is why I would never have ordered that test for you—it's faulty." However, in my case the CA-125 blood tests results were not faulty! My doctor, on the other hand, kept screening me for ovarian cancer. Six months later, I had another transvaginal ultrasound that showed my other ovary to be enlarged. My gynecologist referred me to a gynecologic oncologist for surgery. He found during the surgery that the tumor on my ovaries was ovarian cancer.

It was found early, because my nurse practitioner performed a thorough physical exam, my gynecologist watched me closely and used the CA-125 blood that worked in my case. But that is not what happens to most women with ovarian cancer.

My response to this diagnosis was typical. I was blindsided by it because it was completely unexpected. Although most women are informed of the stage of their ovarian cancer right after they wake up from surgery, I had to wait almost 10 days to find out I was at stage IC. In the meantime, I decided that if ovarian cancer was going to kill me, I wanted to kick it right in the face on the way out! I assumed that like most women in this situation I probably had only a few years to live. I came to this conclusion because I didn't know that a cure was possible since my cancer was discovered early.

In addition to the surgery, I also had six rounds of standard chemotherapy. To date it has been eight years that my cancer has not returned. This was made possible by the early intervention of my nurse practitioner and gynecologist and because my gynecologist referred me to an expert in the field of ovarian cancer surgery—a gynecologic oncologist.

In 1998, I attended the nationwide ovarian cancer conference in Washington, D.C., which was a real turning point for me. A doctor at the conference made a statement that took my breath away. He said that few ovarian cancer activists existed, because women didn't live long enough to become activists. First, I was shocked, then I was angry, and then I realized it was the truth! But despite what that doctor said, I was still convinced that one person could make a big difference. I could already think of people who fit this bill from meeting other ovarian cancer survivors across the country. One of the women who inspired me was Gail Hayward, who founded the National Ovarian Cancer Coalition from her kitchen table.

These days, saving other women from ovarian cancer is my life's work. I spend much of my free time warning women about the threat of this disease, and educating them about risks and interventions. I am concerned that most healthy women do not realize that over 90% of women diagnosed with ovarian cancer have no known prior family history of this disease. I also hear experts say that there could be a biological link between breast and ovarian cancers. Meaning for example, if a woman had breast cancer her chances of getting ovarian cancer also is increased.

I still hold the hope that a better early detection ovarian cancer screening test will become available soon. Although having the CA-125 blood test essentially helped save my life that is not the case for every woman diagnosed with ovarian cancer. Experts think that this test can yield too many false results. In the case of some women with advanced ovarian cancer, the CA-125 results can falsely show no disease. In other cases, it sometimes indicates disease where there is none. Therefore, cancer experts emphasize the need to develop a reliable screening test is essential to detect ovarian cancer early. If we want to detect ovarian cancer early, we need a screening test to be accurate and available to every woman at her annual gynecological exam.

SYMPTOMS ARE OPPORTUNITIES

❖

Ayala

Diagnosed at age 43
In April 2000
With epithelial ovarian cancer
Stage IIIC

Before I was diagnosed with advanced ovarian cancer, I knew nothing about the disease, but I did know that something in my body was not right. Previously, I had been healthy and active with no serious medical problems. When my second son was born, I stopped working as a professional engineer to be a stay-at-home mother. A few years later at 38, I was happily married and a mother of three healthy children, two boys and a girl, ages 9, 6, and 3, fulfilling my life-long dream of having children and a busy family life.

But I started experiencing physical symptoms I never had before. My menstrual cycles were lasting longer, I was getting mid-cycle spotting, vaginal aches, itching, and burning. In the past I had no trouble with my periods, they were always exactly on time and lasted the same length each cycle. When I saw that these symptoms were not going away, I went to my gynecologist (as indicated in my medical records it was in January 1995). I told her about these symptoms, and asked her if they could be due to hormonal changes. She gave me a physical exam and ran some tests. Afterward she told me my hormones were normal but that I had a yeast infection and prescribed a vaginal cream to treat it.

The same uncomfortable symptoms went on until 1996, when I became pregnant with my fourth child. To my surprise and delight, during this pregnancy, all the cycle symptoms and repeated yeast infections disappeared. I was happy to be

11

expecting another child, had a normal pregnancy and delivery, and best of all, a healthy baby boy.

The bleeding that normally lasts for six weeks after a delivery, continued after that period. I called my gynecologist and had vaginal and pelvic ultrasounds. The bleeding stopped shortly after the tests were done, so I did not have to do the D&C procedure, in which the lining of the uterus is scraped—the only thing my doctor had recommended.

The gynecologist didn't tell me that the radiologist (radiology physician) who read these ultrasounds, had noted that there were *"follicular sized ovarian cysts with no evidence of ascites."* Ascites is a fluid that sometimes accumulates in the abdomen with ovarian cancer.

These ultrasounds were done 31/2 years before I was diagnosed with ovarian cancer. Had I known about the cysts, I would have made a considerable effort to seek more information, to know what to do when this condition occur. *Today I know that when symptoms occur and cysts are found, women need to have thorough follow-ups with periodical vaginal ultrasounds, CA-125 blood tests, and complete pelvic examinations including bimanual pelvic exams and recto-vaginal exams in order to make sure the cysts are normal.* If those tests had been administered, from this time on every visit that I had with my gynecologist, I could have been diagnosed with ovarian cancer much sooner.

I never got another vaginal ultrasound, and my doctors did not perform the complete pelvic exam to check my ovaries. They did not check the CA-125. I could find no hint in my medical records that they followed-up on the suspicion the radiologist had that I might have ovarian cancer. This opportunity to have thorough follow-ups was missed. My story presents a critical lesson of why it is important to give complete information regarding test results to patients, even when medical care providers think the results are normal. An informed patient is the best patient, especially when it comes to ovarian cancer. Women can and should seek information by talking to their physicians and asking for copies of their medical tests results.

Unfortunately, I did not ask for my tests results. I was not informed about the ovarian cysts I had at that time despite the fact that they made the radiologist suspect that I might have ovarian cancer.

After the delivery, when my menstrual cycles returned, the symptoms and yeast infections reappeared as before, and I kept complaining about them to my gynecologist. She reassured me everything I experienced was normal and all I needed to do was, to treat the yeast infections. As a result, I had a false sense of security that my symptoms were unrelated to a disease, and concluded that at 40 years old, the yeast infections and cycle symptoms were probably related to peri-menopause or getting older. In addition, since both of my parents were physically fit and healthy, I felt assured of my own good health.

But then I started experiencing a new symptom in my chest. I felt a faint pain in my chest repeatedly when taking deep breaths. The pain seemed to originate from the lowest part of my left lung and was always in the same spot. I had an appointment with my internist about this. He sent me to have a chest X-ray, 15 months before I was diagnosed, and the report indicated that my chest was normal.

All the symptoms up to this point in time were very unpleasant but they did not stop me in my tracks. I appeared healthy and fit. I could persevere and continue to live and function fully even though I was sick with ovarian cancer. However, I became dissatisfied with my medical care and decided that I needed a better gynecologist, hoping to find someone who would be thorough and attentive.

After consulting good friends of mine in the medical community I decided to switch to a new one that they had recommended, and had a routine gynecologic checkup at his office (his notes show it was in February 1999) 14 months before I was diagnosed. I remember feeling very good that day, relived that I finally had found someone I could rely on, and telling him that my main concern was to have thorough medical care in case problems came up in the future. He did a vaginal exam but not a rectal exam and did not ask for my gynecologic medical records.

I then began to have several episodes of sharp pain attacks, what seemed like a nerve pain going through my right shoulder and down my right arm, which intensified when I took deep breaths. 11 months before I was diagnosed, when the pain in my shoulder became severe I called my internist, and the nurse practitioner told me over the phone to take three Advil capsules at once. I followed her orders and the pain went away. I called again when the severe pain recurred. Again, I was blocked by the nurse from talking or seeing the doctor. Her advice was the same—to take three Advil capsules.

In September 1999, 7 months before I was diagnosed, I called my new gynecologist when I experienced severe pelvic pain and spotting. The nurse listened and noted that I was "very upset" but she did not let me speak or see the doctor.

Instead of being a good patient, I should have been a persistent patient and should have insisted on being seen right away. I did not know that the pain I had in my pelvis was another warning sign that I had ovarian cancer. The pain in my shoulder was also serious and I should have insisted on being seen by a doctor for that as well. It is very difficult for me to think about this now. Complaining of symptoms that are warning signs of ovarian cancer was not enough. My health care providers have missed so many opportunities to detect ovarian cancer early and I paid dearly for my unnecessary endurance.

Six months before I was diagnosed, I felt a sharp pain attack in my lower right abdomen, below the rib cage. The pain was so severe that my husband drove me to the emergency room. It was on a late Friday afternoon. We were parked in front of the emergency room about to enter, when my internist called me back on my cell phone. After hearing me describe the symptoms I had over the phone, he told me that it was a gallbladder attack, and said that I should go home. He explained to me that as long as I did not have high fever I should not go to the emergency room. I complied and went home. I checked a medical encyclopedia to find out information about gallbladder attack. He seemed to be right, the pain I felt was located exactly where my gallbladder is supposed to be. I never got a fever and the pain went away over that weekend.

The Monday following this supposed "gallbladder attack" after my pleading, the internist agreed to see me in his office late in the day. He did an external physical exam but no internal exam. The next day an abdominal ultrasound showed my gallbladder to be normal. When I complain to him, that I have been having difficulties getting medical appointments in his office and that his staff was not returning my phone calls, his response was "With $10 co-pays what do you expect." Even though my internist was highly recommended and is considered to be one of the best in my area, after this experience, I began to doubt that my medical care was adequate, and began searching for a new internist.

Five years after my physical symptoms started, I was 43 years old and very busy as a mother taking care of four school-age children. I started to feel more and more fatigued and a little bloated in the abdomen. I had painful periods, gradually over time the abdominal bloating became more severe. On the day I had planned to go to my internist regarding these problems, which was six months after my supposed "gallbladder attack," I awoke with severe abdominal pressure and pain. I could not even wait for his office to open and ended up going to the emergency room instead. A friend drove me there early in the morning on his way to work, while my husband got our children ready for school.

I spent the entire day with my husband in the emergency room, on April 13, 2000, from 7:30 in the morning until 5:00 in the afternoon. I was very lucky that day, the physician running the emergency room was someone we knew. At the end of the day, he concluded that I had diverticulitis and should go home.

As he was getting ready to discharge me, my husband said we needed to find out what was going on before we left the emergency room. My husband's logic was that we could not accept a diagnosis of a problem in the digestive system if none was found. The doctor offered to give me a CAT scan. I did not know what a CAT scan was. I looked at my husband and said that I wanted to go home. He said I should take the scan. I took the scan.

In what seemed like just a few minutes later, several physicians appeared and asked me questions like did I ever have a metal object in my abdomen. I replied no. The emergency room doctor said that the scan showed something suspicious. I was admitted to the hospital and what followed was a whirlwind of tests, and procedures like never before. I was shocked and stunned.

The next morning my doctors came to the hospital and told me I had ovarian cancer, and they introduced me to a gynecologic oncologist for surgery. Four days later, I had a debulking surgery to remove the cancer.

When I read my tests reports, I found out that:

- The scan I had in the emergency room showed "ascites in the pelvis and abdomen and multiple tissue masses within the peritoneum suggestive of peritoneal cancer."

- An abdominal ultrasound showed "the left ovary to be larger than 7 cm."

- A large long needle was inserted into my abdomen and 2 liters of ascites was drained and showed "adenocarcinoma."

- A blood test of CA-125 was 1,684 (35 or less was considered to be normal at that time).

The gynecologic oncologist performed a debulking surgery to remove the cancer, during which the tumor was found to cover the entire surface of my diaphragm. Both my ovaries were affected by the tumor, it was also present in many other areas within the peritoneum. I was diagnosed with advanced epithelial ovarian cancer stage IIIC. A physician also told me that the tumor covering my diaphragm, most likely, was the root cause of the chest pain 15 months prior to the diagnosis, and the sharp nerve pain I experienced in my right shoulder 11 months prior to my ovarian cancer diagnosis.

Before I was diagnosed, I did not realize that all the symptoms I had were related to one illness and in my case meant one thing—ovarian cancer. Like many other ovarian cancer survivors I had additional symptoms. I did not even think they were serious and therefore did not complain to my doctors about them. I had frequent urination, hip pain, lower back aches, shortness of breath and in the last few weeks before I was diagnosed, my bowel movement habits gradually changed, they were getting thinner in size, and I had lost some weight. I did not know that these mere "discomforts" were also ovarian cancer symptoms. I hope that sharing my story will help others know that these kinds of symptoms could potentially be very serious and that good communication between health care providers and patients is important and can lead to early detection of ovarian cancer.

I have had many doctor visits and treatments in the more than four years since I was diagnosed with ovarian cancer. Some of which were:

- A debulking surgery, to remove as much of the cancer as possible.

- Surgery to place a central vein port implant, for chemotherapy.

- Seven cycles of chemotherapy, of Taxol and Carboplatin, administered through this vein port.

- A second look laparoscopy surgery and an intraperitoneal port (IP) put in.

- Second line chemotherapy, through the IP port of 3 cycles of Cisplatin.

- I participated in a phase one clinical trial, in which I received polyvalent vaccines.

- Five more cycles of intravenous chemotherapy of a combination of Carboplatin and Gemcitabine.

I did not expect to be diagnosed with ovarian cancer. I was shocked and felt devastated because I was not going through this alone, my children and my husband were suffering too. Right before my eyes, my life-long dream of a happy family was shattered into pieces by this ovarian cancer storm. I feared that my children might not cope, with such a blow at their young ages—they were only 15, 12, 9, and 31/2 at that time. At times it seemed very bleak, the worst nightmare. I felt trapped and could not see the light at the end of this tunnel.

Despite those feelings, more than four years later, I am still here, in good shape and feeling well. I am happy the emergency room doctor gave me a CAT scan. I credit the efforts and work of the gynecologic oncologists, my medical oncologist, and oncology nurses, with my survival. The love of my family, my husband and children, and the friendship of women survivors I met along my ovarian cancer journey, are a constant help to me.

This disease has challenged our family to adjust to the realities of surviving cancer. My husband and I have put every effort we could to help our children cope through my illness successfully. I think that my children have learned valuable lessons from this traumatic experience. They have grown and become more independent. I feel more assured now that they are stronger, and hope they can overcome whatever the future will bring.

I am thankful for every milestone I am able to take part in. Since I was diagnosed, we have rejoiced in our middle son's Bar Mitzvah and our daughter's Bat Mitzvah. Our oldest son entered college and our youngest son started first grade. I am glad to have realized these milestones, hopes, and dreams. I am looking forward to next year, when our second son will finish his SAT test and applications for college and our daughter will graduate middle school.

On this journey I have learned about ovarian cancer symptoms, treatments, and survival, but I know there is so much more to learn. One of the most valuable lessons that I have learned, and feel compelled to tell others is that every woman knows her body best. She should not overlook or dismiss any symptom. She should persist in pursuing definitive answers when she feels that something in her body is not right, because most likely she is correct. I have learned to keep hopeful, there are ways to cope, and that living with cancer is not as bad as we imagine it to be.

CURED

❖

Mildred

Diagnosed at age 46
In October 1971
With muscinous ovarian cancer
Stage I

I was diagnosed as the result of a biopsy done in the operating room while under general anesthesia. A complete hysterectomy was performed, and the tumor was described as muscinous. I was Stage I ovarian cancer.

While on a vacation, I started feeling ill. One day I felt perfectly fine, the next I felt queasy, had stomach, back, and pelvic pain, frequent urination, and bloating. I was puzzled by what was happening, and felt very uncomfortable so I was determined to see a doctor as soon as I returned home. By the time I reached my last destination, my symptoms became worse, enough to make me want to see a doctor there. I have a low tolerance for pain, and I needed to know what was going on and do something about it. My exam turned out well, but the doctor detected a mass in my abdomen, which he could not explain.

The next day my husband and I flew home, and that afternoon I was in my gynecologist's office. After examining me, he discovered I had a tumor the size of a grapefruit on my right ovary. He was amazed to find it, since he had seen me seven months ago and found nothing there. This gives you some idea of how quickly ovarian cancer grows.

I went to the hospital the next day to have the tumor, which he believed was benign, removed. The day after the surgery, I was taken back to the operating room and in order to wash the interior of my abdomen, I was placed on a rotating table and given what they described as, a radioactive phosphorous treatment through an opening in my abdomen. I had no idea why this was being done. I thought it was part of the whole procedure. I asked no questions, I was so naive then. I simply thought my doctors were doing what was necessary, and once this was finished, I could get on with my life again.

Two years later, I developed thyroid cancer, which I was told was not connected to the ovarian cancer. I survived my second bout with cancer, and continued on, with my life as a wife, mother, and psychotherapist. Each year I went for my checkups and everything was fine.

Fast forward to 22 years later, since I felt so grateful for my survival, that I became interested in volunteering as a way of giving back to other cancer patients. I became involved first at SHARE and later at the Ovarian Cancer National Alliance.

In the meantime, I realized that I knew nothing about my own history. So that year, I went to my annual checkup with many questions. I told my doctor that I was amazed that 22 years had already passed. He made a comment, which astounded me, and revealed something that I had never known before that moment. He said, "I will never forget that morning." Apparently, my tumor had burst that morning. Now I understood why they had taken me back to the operating room for intra peritoneal radiation. If that treatment had not been successful, I would not be here today. It was then that I learned about my stage and tumor type. I was shocked and astounded that I had never known how serious the situation had been at the time. And if I had never asked, I still wouldn't know to this day.

How have I coped with having cancer twice? Initially, I continued to live my life the same way I did before I was diagnosed. I was a strong believer in a healthy diet, which I practiced more assiduously than ever. After my initial questions about how this could have happened to me, despite my good nutrition and the fact that I took good care of myself, I realized that my family history had played a role. There were several cancer deaths in my immediate family, and it was possible that I was on that genetic line. Because I am the only cancer survivor in my family, I like to think my strong immune system and healthy diet played an important part in my survival. Other things that helped me get through it are very good psychotherapy, an active work life, and a supportive family. Most importantly, becoming involved in the ovarian cancer movement and making a contribution there, has given me the biggest boost for my own healing and well-being.

Knowing that I speak out for the need for early detection of ovarian cancer, and working with women who are currently facing the disease, has enriched my life tremendously. Working towards the goal of helping other women has given me the greatest gift. I feel extremely privileged to be involved with such important work.

PERSISTANCE PAYS

✦

Judy

Diagnosed at age 55
In March 2000
With Mullerian ovarian cancer
Stage IIB

I am a wife, mother, daughter, sister, aunt, friend, and social worker. I am also an ovarian cancer survivor.

In March 2000, I was very happy and healthy. I also felt content and lucky in my life. I was 55 years old, happily married for 34 years. My grown children were at good places in their lives. My daughter had just received her master's degree and my son had just become engaged. I had just returned from a short trip to Florida, visiting my parents who were in good health and very independent. I had recently changed careers, returning to social work after more than 20 years in business, and I loved my job as administrator of a geriatric mental health clinic and director of a social program for people with dementia.

My health, aside from orthopedic aches and pains, was excellent. I woke up each day energized and excited that I was making a contribution in a field I loved. I was on hormone-replacement therapy for osteoporosis, and monitored closely, seeing my gynecologist every six months. I had regular mammograms each year and believed I was conscientious in taking charge of my own body. What I did not know, was that a malignant tumor was growing in my ovary.

On Friday March 17, St. Patrick's Day, my children joined my husband and me for dinner. I served corned beef and cabbage, a meal I cook each year on the holiday. Each year we always comment on how much we enjoy this meal and wonder why I only prepare it once a year. However, that evening, I was unable to eat more than a few mouthfuls. I complained that my stomach was upset, nothing major, but I was feeling a little achy. For the rest of the weekend, my lower abdomen continued to bother me.

When I awoke on Monday, I mentioned to my husband that I still felt "funny" and noticed that I felt pressure when I needed to urinate. Thinking it could have been a urinary tract infection, I decided to call my doctor. I debated whether to call my gynecologist or my internist. I chose to call my internist, who I had been seeing for 20 years. He was also a gastroenterologist, and I thought my problem was related to his field of expertise. Not for one moment, did I suspect that I had cancer. Cancer was something that happened to other people in other families.

I called my doctor from my office that Monday morning, and his staff told me that he was very busy that week, and since it was not an emergency, they could fit me in that Friday. I insisted that I had to see him that day. I often wondered why I was so demanding, I attributed it to believing I had an infection, and thinking that the sooner I got on antibiotics, the better. I requested that the staff asked my doctor if he would see me, and they gave me an appointment for noon that same day. I later asked my doctor why he agreed to see me the same day, he responded that since he had never seen me act so concerned, he wanted to accommodate me.

My doctor performed a complete examination including a vaginal and rectal exam, something he had never done in the past. He asked me many questions regarding my symptoms, and took an X-Ray of my abdomen. He said it did not look like I had a urinary tract infection, but the X-ray indicated that I might have diverticulitis. He scheduled a CAT scan of my abdomen and pelvis the next day. In retrospect, I was totally oblivious to any concern he was feeling regarding my health, and asked if I could take the tests a few days later, since I was very busy, but he said he wanted it done the next day, so he could have the results that Thursday.

After I had the CAT scan, the technician and radiologist did not tell me anything, only that my doctor would call me with the results. I was not alarmed. For the next day and a half, I went to work. Although my stomachache had intensified a bit, I attributed it to the unpleasant solution I had to drink for my scan.

When I spoke to my doctor on Thursday, he stated that he wanted my husband and me to come in to talk to him the next day. I asked him what was the matter, and he responded that he preferred to talk to us in person. I insisted that he tell me my results over the phone, and he said that the CAT scan showed a large pelvic mass that was probably ovarian cancer. It is hard to describe the feeling that came over me. I can only compare it to the feeling I had on Sept 11 when I watched the second plane hit the building. I knew it was true, but at the same time, I could not believe this was happening to me. I asked him if it could have been a benign cyst and he said it was possible, but unlikely given its characteristics. He then told me that we could treat it, and that he would be with us each step of the way. I hung up the phone and called my husband giving him the horrible news of how our lives had changed forever. Although he was devastated, he remained my "tower of strength" throughout this ordeal.

The next day we saw our doctor. He greeted us with the warmest of hugs. We told him that I wanted to do whatever it took to beat this. How did I get it? What had I done for this to happen? He answered our questions, reassuring us that I would receive the best possible treatment. Although this was very serious, he believed that I could win this battle.

My doctor sent me to a gynecologic oncologist. I had never even heard of this specialty. He spent over an hour talking to my husband and me. More tests were scheduled before surgery could be done. I was scheduled for a radical hysterectomy along with staging (diagnosis of the stage of cancer), in order to remove as much of the tumor as possible. He told me I would need chemo, and that the next six months would be "very hard work." I told him that I had never been afraid of hard work. He made it clear that I could beat this, and that a cure was possible.

After surgery, the gynecologic oncologist reported that although the tumor was large, he believed he had removed all of it, and there were no visible signs of any remaining tumor. The results of the pathology tests yielded both good and bad news. The good news was that there was not any lymph node involvement, and my fluids were clean. The bad news was that my tumor was unusual. I had a malignant mixed mesodermal or mullerian tumor. There was no standard treatment for it. He also told us that it would be devastating to read literature about this kind of tumor, which is usually seen at late stages of cancer when treatment has not been successful. He told us to disregard all of that. My case was different, since it was found early, and could be treated. He assured us that he and his colleagues would do copious research and consult with other doctors to devise my customized treatment. My treatment would be very aggressive, we were going for the cure.

We also went for a second opinion, and that oncologist not only concurred with my doctor, but he indicated that he would speak with my doctor to help find the appropriate course of treatment.

I received six cycles of Cisplatin and Ifosfamide, each session required me to stay in the hospital from Monday to Friday. It was difficult, but I was never very sick. I experienced some nausea, loss of appetite, hair loss, and fatigue after the third cycle. I then had 25 days of pelvic radiation, an unusual treatment for ovarian cancer, but one that has been successful when a mullerian tumor occurs in the uterus. My radiation oncologist also was extremely positive that I was going to beat this.

Since finishing treatment, I have been cancer free with low CA-125 numbers and no evidence of disease on my CAT scans. I feel healthy once again and blessed that my cancer was diagnosed so early. I often wonder what made me go to my doctor as quickly as I did and why he took the time to listen to my symptoms, and recognized the possibility that it could be ovarian cancer. I will always be thankful for that, and I believe that he and my excellent, skilled surgeon saved my life.

But most women with ovarian cancer are not as lucky as I was. Many, like my friend Cynthia, who died just a year after diagnosis, go to the doctor with bloating, abdominal pain, and bowel disturbances. GI tests may be run but if they come back negative, they are often told that nothing is wrong, that their symptoms are due to stress or depression. Months later, many of these women find out that they now have advanced ovarian cancer. I try to pass this message on to medical students, to remember this so that when a woman comes to them with similar symptoms, they can one day be thankful that they saved her life.

MY CHANCES OF GETTING OVARIAN CANCER

❖

Wendy

Diagnosed at age 50
In January 2000
With ovarian cancer
Stage IIIC

On Jan 20, 2004, 29 years to the day had passed since my mother died from ovarian cancer, when she was 60, and I was 25. My mother was a very private person, she did not tell anyone, neither family nor friends, what type of cancer she had. It was only in my forties that I got a copy of her death certificate and learned that she had died of ovarian cancer. A year after she died, my maternal aunt died, on the same day, of breast cancer at the age of 70.

I told my gynecologist about my mother and aunt, and that I had another aunt who had breast cancer as well as a cousin who died from breast cancer at the age of 41. He told me not to worry about it, and that my chances of getting ovarian cancer were no greater than anyone else's. However, I insisted on having an ultrasound done every year. I wanted a CA-125 blood test done every year, but he said that it was not accurate, and that I should not have it done.

In 1998, I started to have a pain in my stomach whenever I ate. My doctor sent me to a gastroenterologist. I told her about my mother, but she just ignored it. I had every test done, and nothing showed up positive. She said I had irritable bowel syndrome.

I had heard about genetic testing being done for diseases, and went to a meeting about it. I was going to have a blood test done to see if I had the gene for breast and ovarian cancer, but my gynecologist told me not to do the genetic testing. He said the hospital was doing the testing to get money from the government.

In December 1999, the pain in my stomach became unbearable. I went to the gastroenterologist and she just said if the pain got any worse to go to the emergency room. I knew that something was really wrong. On that same day, I went to see my gynecologist and had an ultrasound done, which revealed a small cyst. He said it was not big enough to cause me any pain, and that he would do another ultrasound in six weeks.

When I had the second ultrasound done, the cyst had grown to the size of an orange. My doctor called and said he wanted me to have a CAT scan done right away. The scan showed something on my other ovary.

I made an appointment with a gynecologic oncologist and within a week, I was in the hospital having surgery. During the surgery, they found that I had advanced ovarian cancer stage IIIC.

I was given three options for treatment after surgery. I chose the most aggressive treatment, which was chemotherapy with stem-cell replacement therapy. First, I had my stem cells removed. Then I was hospitalized and received strong chemotherapy for three days. On the fourth day, I had some of my own stem cells replaced. I did this four times. The fourth time I developed an infection and went into a coma. When I came out of it, I was so weak I could not walk or talk. I had to go into a physical rehab for two weeks. Then I had another surgery to make sure the cancer was gone.

I have since found out that I have the gene suspected for ovarian cancer. I have two daughters. They have been tested and we are waiting for the results.

UNPREDICTABLE GENETICS

❖

Lisa

Diagnosed at age 42
In September 1999
With ovarian cancer
Stage IIIC

During the past three and a half years, I have survived ovarian cancer twice.

I knew about cancer from the time my aunt passed away from breast cancer at a young age, and my mother's breast cancer forced her to have a mastectomy right before my wedding. Following my mother's battle with cancer, I have been mindful that breast cancer ran in my family, and went for checkups and mammograms regularly. In addition to that, I was always very good about eating a healthy diet and exercising regularly to help decrease my chances of getting cancer.

In September 1999, I was diagnosed with Stage IIIC ovarian cancer and my world was turned upside down. Unfortunately, my doctors did not realize that I was exhibiting symptoms of ovarian cancer long before my diagnosis.

Just a month before, I went to a general practitioner complaining of fatigue, bloating, and that my stomach just did not feel right. He diagnosed me with IBS (Irritable Bowel Syndrome). He prescribed Donnatol and sent me on my way, without even giving me a physical exam. Needless to say, the medication did not help and I started feeling worse.

Labor Day weekend that year was the turning point for me. My period became irregular, which led me to believe that my problem was gynecological. My suspicion was correct—After seeing a gynecologist, I was diagnosed with ovarian cancer, and soon after had surgery.

All of my doctors knew about my family's history of breast cancer, but not one of them explained to me that I had an increased risk of developing ovarian cancer as well. I now know that experts believe the two forms of cancer can have a common genetic link. When my symptoms started, my doctors did not suggest that I undergo a vaginal ultrasound, which would have been an appropriate measure.

I believe that if my doctors had advised me to have vaginal ultrasound tests, they would have been able to diagnose my disease earlier, when the stage of ovarian cancer could have been lower, and chances for long survival better. I feel strongly about this issue and that doctors should advise their patients to take this test, as soon as they complain of similar problems. Since my experience, I have urged my friends who have similar symptoms to ask their doctors for vaginal ultrasound tests.

After I had the surgery, and most of the cancer was debulked (removed), I underwent chemotherapy with a combination of Taxol and Carboplatin. The road ahead was difficult. I was living in a state of disbelief. Wondering how this could have happened to me and became worried of my own mortality. I never recovered from the state of shock that set in after the diagnosis. I was terrified of dying all the time. I felt bad enough to seek psychological help and received anti-depressants. During that time, my husband and I tried to educate ourselves to the best of our ability about the disease, to prepare ourselves for the road that lay ahead of us.

I was in remission for the two years, but had a recurrence in September 2001. The chemotherapy was difficult and exhausting the second time around, but I managed to get through it. After completing the chemotherapy, I participate in a Phase II clinical trial of anti-cancer medications. In this study I and received two drugs thought to inhibit the growth of cancer cells. One was Casodex, a prostate cancer drug that I took daily. The second was Luprin, which was administered as a shot under the skin of the abdomen once a month.

The second chemotherapy treatments worked, and to date, December 2003 I am still in remission. I feel lucky that chemotherapy has worked twice, and to have the support network, of family and friends, to help me fight this battle.

Unfortunately, my immune system was extremely weakened from the chemotherapy treatments. I had to quit my job as a teacher's aid for children in special education to devote more time to my own care. I often joke that my current full-time job is taking care of myself instead of children. I try to keep one step ahead, by being physically fit, and seeing my doctors regularly.

Another thing I am focusing on these days, is educating myself about genetic testing. This topic is important to me, since I have two young daughters. When they are old enough, I plan on having them tested to see if they are at risk for ovarian and breast cancer.

The results of my genetic testing indicated a possible genetic link to ovarian cancer, surprisingly on my father's side of the family. Yet in his family, there is no history of ovarian cancer and longevity is prevalent. My case is an example of how unpredictable genetics can be. As a protective measure, my older daughter is currently taking birth control pills, because physicians believe that taking them might reduce the chances of developing ovarian cancer.

Although it seems at times that I have everything under control, my struggle with this dreadful disease will stay with me for the rest of my life. I recently lost a dear friend from my ovarian cancer support group. Losing a close friend from this disease adds to the anxiety I have about my future. Even closer to home, my sister was also diagnosed with ovarian cancer after my own battle with the disease started. Unfortunately, she was not as lucky as I was. Her system resisted the chemotherapy treatments and she passed away recently, at the age of 51.

My method of coping with this grief is to try to do whatever I can to make a difference in the lives of cancer patients. Along with my husband, friends, and family, I contribute and fundraise as much as I can for ovarian cancer awareness and research.

MY JUNIOR PROM DRESS

✦

Krissy

Diagnosed at age 17
In May 1997
With ovarian cancer endodermal sinus
Stage IC

Seven years ago, in the spring of 1997, I began having pains in my abdomen. These pains were like no other stomachache or cramp I had ever felt in my life. I was 17 years old. My dad had recently been diagnosed with bladder cancer. I thought these pains could have been caused by an ulcer I contracted from worrying about him. At first, I did not tell my parents because I didn't want them worrying about me. My dad was going through enough already. Soon after the pains started, I began gaining weight quickly, and it seemed like the weight was only going to my stomach area. As odd as it may sound, I did not associate the pain with the weight gain. My junior prom was approaching, and I could barely fit into the dress I had bought only two months before. Finally on Wednesday after the prom, I told my mom that I really thought I should go to the doctor.

Since it is unlike me to make such a request, my mom knew something was wrong and got an appointment for me to see the family doctor that afternoon. My doctor asked me questions then insisted I was pregnant. After I assured him that it was not possible, he took an X-Ray, which revealed a number of dark spots. My doctor was puzzled by the results. He repeatedly asked me if I had eaten anything out of the ordinary that day, and if I was certain I had taken all metallic objects off my body before taking the X-Ray. He then did a pap smear, which at the age of seventeen was terrifying since I did not have this examination done before, and all of a sudden I was being thrown into it.

He concluded that I had an ovarian cyst, and that I should not be alarmed since these are very common. My mom, having my dad constantly in mind, specifically asked if it could be cancer. My doctor laughed and said "No." He ordered an ultrasound, and explained that if the cyst was smaller than a grapefruit we could treat it with medication, but if it was larger then I would need to have surgery to remove it.

Friday, two days later, an ultrasound showed this "cyst" to be the size of a football. My dreaded surgery was scheduled for Tuesday, four days later. My doctor explained to me that I would have to miss my prom, as he feared dancing could cause this huge cyst to pop. When I told him I had already attended it the previous weekend, he almost fainted!

From Friday through that weekend, my pain and abdomen size intensified so much that my physical movements became severely restricted. I could not sit, stand, or lay, it all hurt too much. By Sunday, which ironically was Mother's Day, I looked like a nine-month pregnant teen about to give birth. Because this "cyst" was growing so rapidly, they admitted me into surgery right away on Monday morning, on the same day that my dad had his first cancer treatment.

A gynecologist performed my surgery, on May 12 1997. The operation revealed a surprise to her—this so-called "cyst" was indeed ovarian cancer. My family was told there was an unexpected occurrence, and that the surgery would last a while longer. The gynecologist carefully removed the large fifteen-pound malignant tumor, which was growing on my right ovary and expanded across towards my left ovary. In addition to the tumor, she removed my right ovary and fallopian tube, lymph nodes, and surrounding tissue. I remember immediately after waking up from surgery, having the sensation of my stomach being gone and empty, it felt like it was sunken in.

One of the two oncologists in my hometown was assigned to me. He worked directly with my gynecologist in my treatment. I got a second opinion at a university medical center, where they agreed with my doctors' diagnosis that the tumor was a malignant endodermal sinus tumor (a subtype germ cell malignant tumor) and that I needed chemotherapy.

I underwent a summer of intense chemotherapy, in which I received three cycles of Bleomyacin, Cysplatnum, and Etopacide. My treatments were on an outpatient basis. Each cycle lasted from 8 a.m. to 4 p.m., Monday through Friday for the first week, and only on Mondays for the following two weeks. I was followed up with blood tests of alpha feta protein cancer marker, which at surgery was over 1,200 (under 15 being considered normal). After surgery, it was cut in half, and for the most part I continued to respond well to the chemo, bringing my cancer markers down almost every time I had treatment.

As with most cancer patients, I had many setbacks and suffered many side effects. Including hair loss, mouth and throat sores, dark skin discoloration, seizure-like symptoms from Compazine an anti-nausea medication. I also developed Raynaud Syndrome, a circulatory condition that I will have for the rest of my life, but I believe it is a small price to pay for survival. Losing my hair was not too hard for me, because my friends and family constantly made a joke of it. My sister would always bring me new hats and bandanas. My uncle bought me a shirt that said, "With a body like this, who needs hair!" My brother would even draw life-like faces on the back of my head! To me, all these were better than wearing a wig!

Now, at the age of twenty-four, I go for check-ups once a year. I call it "the week from hell," because I have to take so many tests and I have so much anxiety about them. However, I am confident that with my thorough check-ups, if anything were to come up again, it would be caught early.

Like all other young survivors I have met, I also heard many people say that I was too young for this to happen to me, which is neither comforting nor true. All of us were told this by not only friends, families, and people in the community, but also by our doctors. *The reality is that a woman of any age can get ovarian cancer.*

Looking back, I am fortunate to have had strong enough symptoms to make surgery necessary, which subsequently led to my correct and early diagnosis of ovarian cancer. If it had not been for that, I might have been misdiagnosed numerous times, as this happens to so many women with ovarian cancer.

As horrible as this disease is, I would never trade my experience. That is starting to sound like a cliché coming from survivors, but it is true. In addition to bringing my family closer together and making my Christian faith stronger, my experience allowed me to meet so many amazing people that I otherwise would have never met. It also guided me to a career choice in public health education. Among other things, I realize how precious life really is, and I look forward to continuing that circle with my own family someday, which I am so blessed I still am able to do.

A BIRTHDAY MESSAGE OF
SURVIVAL

❖

Sharon

Diagnosed at age 42
In February 1995
With ovarian cancer
Stage IIC

If someone asked me the question if cancer ever ends, sadly enough I would have to say no. It seems that every time I turn around, I hear about someone being diagnosed with cancer, facing a recurrence, or dying. But let's not forget, we often hear about people surviving cancer for a long time. I like those stories, and I need to hear them, so that is why I have written mine. It is also a birthday message, as I just celebrated my 52nd birthday in February 2004, which nine years ago, I was not sure that I would be around to do.

The short history of my ovarian cancer journey is as follows. I was diagnosed in February 1995 with Stage IIC Ovarian cancer, probably epithelial, at the age of 42. I had experienced pelvic pain for about three months, so my gynecologist sent me to have a transvaginal ultrasound, which revealed an enlarged right ovary.

I celebrate two anniversary dates, the first being February 7 when I was diagnosed with ovarian cancer during a laparoscopy surgery. The second is February 11when I had emergency surgery—the big TAH-BSO (Total Abdominal Hysterectomy—Bilateral Salpingo Oophorectomy) due to a ruptured appendix and a nasty case of periotonitis. I have a big scar down my middle, instead of a neatly stitched scar line, that was left to close up on its own due to the risk of infection from the appendicitis. When asked which one is the actual date of my life being saved, I tell people that I celebrate both.

I had six rounds of Taxol and Carboplatin through a port. I have thankfully remained free of disease since I finished treatment in July 1995. A year or so after my initial surgery, I did have a partial bowel obstruction—the worst pain I'd ever had. To treat it, I had a cantor tube procedure. A tube with a bag filled with mercury was pushed down my nose and peristalsis pulled the bag down into the area of the obstruction, attempting to clear it. Thankfully, after 10 days in the hospital, it did the trick for me. It would not have worked if I had a tumor, and I do not think this procedure is widely used anymore, but I might be wrong. The worst part of the procedure was the removal of the tube, but I survived to tell the tale. I have many adhesions due to my surgery and the appendicitis. My doctor told me that they would eventually "settle down." Thankfully, I have not had problems since my partial bowel obstruction.

There are several steps I took in order to get through it all, and arrive at this place where I am now. The first was joining SHARE, an ovarian support group in New York City to find other women with this disease. Back in 1995, there was not a whole lot of information or support available, and I felt so relieved to be able to talk and ask questions of these other women, who were farther along in the process of the disease. I also signed onto the Ovarian Problems Discussion Listserv in December 1995, when it had around 75 subscribers (it currently has about 1,200) and met many amazing folks there over the years, some of them in person. Of course, I received "Conversations" an ovarian cancer survivor's news letter that is also available on the web. Cindy Melancon, its founder, was an amazing woman. I also met Gail Hayward, the founder of NOCC (National Ovarian Coalition) who served as another inspiration for me when I needed one. I was around to watch the beginnings of the ovarian cancer movement the founding of OCNA (Ovarian Cancer National Alliance) for example. The first OCNA conference was an incredible experience, with so many of us bursting out of the hotel conference room, the air charged with excitement that we were all gathered together to try to make a difference in getting the word out about this disease.

I went on to facilitate a support group for several years, did volunteer hotline work, helped to organize a memorial quilt program at my hospital, and became involved with several other projects. As time passed though, I found that I needed to get back to doing what I loved to do—concentrating on my art. I'm a professional painter dealing with the never ending struggle of trying to make a living and survive as an artist, which is not an easy feat. Although I am not as active as I once was in helping others with the disease, I am still active in that arena, and help other newly diagnosed women in whatever ways I can. And I know that there are others like me who are long-term survivors who quietly go about their lives and work "behind the scenes" to help others dealing with this disease. They are out there—women can and do survive ovarian cancer.

THANKS TO THE RADIOLOGIST

◆

Kristen

Diagnosed at age 38
In August 2003
With ovarian cancer
Stage IIIC

I am an ovarian cancer survivor. Since I had no symptoms, my annual gynecological exam saved my life. In early June 2003, my gynecologist detected a lump on my right ovary. In mid June, a vaginal ultrasound revealed a mass. Since my gynecologist did not perform surgery, I was referred to another doctor in the practice, which resulted in a two-week delay before I had surgery. An MRI was done in the beginning of July and the next day, I was told the mass was suspicious of cancer and there was excess fluid in my abdomen. So I was referred to a gynecologic oncologist.

I thought to myself that there was no way the mass on my ovary was cancerous. I felt fine and had no symptoms. I ate a healthy diet and got plenty of exercise, as I had been a long distance runner for years.

I called the oncologist's office and took the next available appointment, which was two months later. I sent all prior test results to the oncologist and was instructed to schedule a pelvic and abdominal CAT scan and CA-125 blood test. I did not feel worried, and thought that I had plenty of time to schedule these tests. Lo and behold, when I got home from work that day, there was a message from the oncologist's office changing my appointment from two months away to only two weeks away.

I remember thinking that this must be serious. My gynecologist must have called the oncologist and raised a red flag. Two weeks later, when I met with the oncologist, he revealed that the CAT scan echoed the MRI results and my CA-125 blood test was normal. The CA-125 never worked for me, the results were always 13, even when I had advanced ovarian cancer.

The mass on the right ovary had to be removed and tested. My gynecological oncologist scheduled my surgery for one month later and ordered several additional tests, an MRI of my liver and a barium enema of my colon. The barium enema was sub-optimal and a colonoscopy was done, which came out clear.

My attitude remained positive as I felt that there was no way I had cancer. I was 38 at the time, which I felt was too young to have cancer, healthy and physically fit. I had no symptoms. How could I possibly have had cancer? I ran 3 to 5 miles a day and practiced Tae Kwon Do twice a week. And cancer did not run in my family. I didn't tell anyone that there was a possibility I had cancer prior to my surgery. I didn't want to consider the mass cancerous until it was taken out and tested.

Nervous and not knowing what to expect, I prepared for surgery. I was sick and tired of the endless testing. I wanted all of this behind me to be able to move on with my life.

I woke up in the recovery room wondering what had happened to me. The nurses told me the doctor would be in to explain. I dozed on and off, but kept wondering what had happened during the surgery. I noticed the clock on the wall read 2:00 p.m. I remember thinking to myself that I had been in the operating room for a long time and that the tumor must have been cancerous.

A few hours later, in a hospital room I tracked down my husband. I asked him what happened and he told me the news: The tumor was malignant and the cancer had spread to my left ovary and abdomen. The doctors had performed a radical hysterectomy and debulking procedure. Various biopsies had been taken and sent to two different pathology labs for evaluation.

I could not believe what I heard, nothing seemed real. I focused all my energy on recovering from the surgery. Everyone who heard the news was stunned. Gifts, flowers, and cards poured into my home. People were distressed, but all along, I kept telling everyone that I was fine. The surgery was a success and since I was in good health, the incision was small and healed well. I did not understand why everyone was so worried. They acted as if I received my death sentence. I began to wonder if I was not taking my situation seriously enough.

Two weeks after the surgery my oncologist reviewed the pathology results and revealed that, I had Stage IIIC ovarian cancer. I was prescribed six chemotherapy treatments of a combination of Taxol/Carboplatin taken at 21-day intervals. About a month after surgery, my chemotherapy treatment began. I received a tour of the chemotherapy area at the hospital and tons of information. I read up about it non-stop, and spoke to anyone that I could about ovarian cancer. However, the irony was I still did not associate myself with the disease. It was as if I was learning about it for someone else's benefit.

When my first treatment was scheduled, I cut off 12 inches of my long hair to make my hair loss seem less traumatic. I was very anxious about losing my hair and made endless appointments to be fitted for wigs, as I did not think that hats and scarves were for me. I felt that they drew attention to an individual and screamed "cancer patient." I bought one wig prior to my first chemo treatment.

Twenty-four hours before the treatment, I had to take a steroid called Decadron to help me tolerate the drugs. I was very nervous, the thought of these toxic chemicals being in my body made me sick to my stomach.

The first treatment was run at a slower rate to allow the doctors to monitor for adverse reactions. All of the chemo drugs were delivered intravenously. The following premedications were administered: Kytril and Decadron for anti nausea, Tagamet as a stomach protectorant and Benadryl to prevent allergic reactions. Next was the Taxol, I could feel it moving through my veins, and it filled my body with strange sensations. I became very fidgety and emotional. I cried at the thought of these chemicals running through me. I told myself over and over again that chemo was good for me and it was meant to clean out the cancerous cells. The final drug of the session was the Carboplatin.

The doctor and nurses checked on me constantly and assured me that I was tolerating the drugs well. My chemo sessions took six to seven hours on average. Each time, I was sent home with a shot of Neulasta to be given 24 hours after treatment to boost my white cell count, along with a drug called Zofran to take twice a day for the next four days to help with nausea. My blood levels were checked 10 days later, following each session. Typically, I was given a shot of Aranesp to boost my red cell count in preparation for the next round of chemo, which would be 11 days later.

With each treatment, my fatigue and nausea increased. After my first treatment, I had a lot of difficulty sleeping and felt very sad and emotional. In addition, I was very anxious about losing my hair. About 10 days after my first treatment, I noticed that I was losing more hair in the shower. I immediately made an appointment to get my haircut even shorter, this time "Boy short", to make my baldness feel less traumatic. I even decided not to wash my hair in hopes that it would not disappear. Unfortunately, the next day more hair disappeared, and when I got home from work and took off my coat off my collar was full of hair. I said to my daughter that my coat looked like a porcupine. My daughter told me that it was all over the back of my dress. I was completely devastated. I did not know what to do.

Maybe I really was convinced that this was not going to happen to me, and now, with my hair falling out, I got a reality check. I got into the shower and felt the water washing my hair away. In tears, I got out of the shower thinking there could not possibly be any more hair left on my head. I still had some hair, but I had bald patches everywhere. I wrapped a towel around my head, and my husband called friends of ours that own a salon to see if they could shave my head. I went to the salon first thing the next morning to have my head shaved. I left the salon wearing my wig and feeling very strange. The wig did not feel natural, but surprisingly I was OK with my baldness. I ended up purchasing some hats and scarves and only wore the wig to work.

Some of the unexpected side effects from the chemotherapy were muscle pain and neuropathy (nerve damage). About five days following each treatment, I would get severe muscle pain in my legs. It went away after a few days, however, the neuropathy was a different story. I have developed neuropathy in my hands and feet. This condition causes a feeling of pins and needles, tingling, burning, and numbness. The more stimulation my nervous system gets, the more likely I will have pain in my hands, feet, and occasionally scalp. The more time I spend on my feet and the more I do with my hands, the more apt I am to have a neuropathy attack. The pain gets so intense, that I go out of my mind. This condition prevents me from doing things like walking for any length of time, physical exercise, and housework, which I guess could be viewed as a good thing. It also prevents me from going out, since I never know when I will get an attack and when this happens, I do not feel comfortable being around other people.

There are no short cuts, I am taking my recovery one day at a time, and I do my best to remain positive. At one point, I just wanted my life to return to the way it was prior to surgery, but I realize that I am not that same person. Cancer has changed my life. Cancer has been an experience. I have learned more about myself and others. I have gained insight into my fears, strengths, and concerns. Cancer is a full-time job. Dealing with doctors, treatments, and various medical procedures can consume a lot of time and energy. But I try to remain positive and live life to its fullest, while undergoing all the necessary tests, procedures, and treatments.

It is also important to have a good relationship with your doctors. My oncologist is fabulous. He is an excellent surgeon who has an excellent bedside manner. He always keeps me informed about my treatment and takes time to answer my questions and explain the answers in layman's terms. I thanked him for doing his job extremely well, and I am very grateful that the tumor was removed so quickly.

I asked why my appointment had been moved ahead two months, and he told me the radiologist doctor at the imaging center, called him expressing urgency with what he saw on the X-rays. Who knows how much further advanced my cancer would have been if this call had not been made?

It is important for doctors to diagnose thoroughly patient's symptoms. It is equally important for patients not to ignore common symptoms, and for women never to skip their annual gynecologic exam.

I was lucky that my doctor found my ovarian cancer when I had no apparent symptoms, however most women do have symptoms, which unfortunately are not recognized as early as they should be. Some common symptoms of ovarian cancer are abnormal bleeding, backaches, bloating, constipation, exhaustion, frequent urination, indigestion, intestinal gas, and shortness of breath.

There are no guarantees when it comes to life, and no bias or discrimination when it comes to cancer.

NOT A PULLED MUSCLE

◆

Kathy

Diagnosed at age 51
In February 2002
With epithelial ovarian cancer
Stage III

In August 2001, I was having a great summer. I was playing golf regularly, although perhaps not scoring as well as I wanted. I was involved in a very exciting consulting project for my job, and enjoying the fifth year of married life. I went to my gynecologist for my annual check-up, something I was careful about doing each year, and everything was fine. I told my doctor that I was having some discomfort during intercourse, and she assured me it was just dryness due to peri-menopause.

That September was very stressful because of the World Trade Center attacks. I was living only a few blocks away from the site, I saw the planes strike and the buildings collapse, and was displaced from my work site for over a week.

By early October, I noticed a pain in my lower left abdomen. I noticed it the most when I was doing sit-ups or when I was riding the exercise bicycle. I did not pay much attention to it though, because I assumed it was a result of a combination of stress from 9/11, and repercussions of my vigorous exercise routine.

By the end of October, I noticed the pain was increasing a bit, and my pants fit tighter. I was feeling bloated and nauseous. I assumed that this was stress-related.

In November, I went for an examination from my primary-care physician who thought I had a pulled muscle. He told me to stop doing sit-ups and to schedule another appointment if it was not better in a few weeks.

My abdominal pain and bloating grew more acute. The nausea started being accompanied by a shortness of breath, which occurred from time-to-time, but not consistently. In fact, during the holiday season, I noticed the pain had not subsided, and that there was a lump in that same area of my abdomen where I was experiencing pain. Rather than go back to my regular doctor, I self-diagnosed that something might have been wrong with my colon and scheduled a colonoscopy.

The gastroenterologist talked with me at length about my symptoms, and gave me an internal physical exam. I have to say, that I was very impressed that he spent a lot of time talking to me about my symptoms. After the exam, he did blood-work and told me to schedule a CAT scan, which I slated for mid-Feb, 2002.

I was told that the results of the CAT scan and my symptoms were consistent with ovarian cancer. I felt like I was having a bad dream. I heard what the doctor said, but could not believe it. I left his office in a state of shock. I can remember standing on 14th Street, calling my husband on my cell phone, crying. The doctor sent one of his staff members after me to ask if they could accompany me home. I got home in a daze.

My internist referred me to a gynecologic oncologist whom I went to see the next day. He confirmed that I had Stage 3 epithelial ovarian cancer and recommended surgery as soon as possible. I appreciated the forthright way he explained everything about the cancer, and what to expect during the surgery. I went home and spent a lot of time preparing my advanced directives, and reading Buddhist texts on death and dying. I had never had surgery, and felt simultaneously terrified and hopeful.

The surgery was long, about seven hours. They removed everything except my uterus including my ovaries, fallopian tubes, omentum, and various miscellaneous tumors and, in an unexpected development, a large section of my bowel. So I woke up from surgery being a cancer survivor with a colostomy. That was one of the most difficult parts of dealing with the diagnosis of cancer. Not only did I have to deal with having cancer, but also I had to deal with the lifestyle change that having a colostomy brings. I spent the first few days after the surgery asking the question "why me?" I detested myself. I felt as though the life as I knew it had ended. Fortunately, both oncologists that had operated on me assured me that the colostomy was temporary and that after chemotherapy I could have the procedure reversed. And even more fortunately, I had a wonderful ostomy nurse who guided me through several weeks after the surgery and beyond.

The surgery was pronounced successful: they had done the maximum debulking of the tumors. I had six rounds of chemotherapy, Carboplatin and Taxol.

The recovery from each round of chemotherapy was difficult. I continued to work, I only missed a total of three to four days throughout the chemotherapy, but I really felt debilitated and demoralized with my inability to function effectively at home and at work.

The lessons I have learned from Buddhism have kept me going. That we should take one day at a time, since all we have is now. We cannot change the past, or predict the future. And to recognize that we only suffer when we resist what life has dealt us, or long for what we don't have.

I had surgery in late October to restore my bowel function. At the same time, my doctor finished my hysterectomy, performed an appendectomy, and removed one small tumor.

After multiple consultations and much careful thought, I decided, in conjunction with my medical oncologist, not to undergo a second round of chemotherapy at that time, electing instead to take Tamoxifen. The result of my March 2003 CA-125 was 4 (which is within the normal range). A CAT scan I had taken one month later, found the presence of four additional tumors. The CA-125 blood test is not a good marker for me. Despite having advanced cancer, my count was only in the mid-200s.

So, needless to say, I was devastated. I went through a period of feeling very depressed, convinced that I would become a bad statistic of ovarian cancer. But I'm back in chemotherapy, pursuing complementary therapies and researching what options I might have in the future if this round doesn't work.

Recently, I thought back to my gynecologic exam in August 2001. I realized that I do not think she gave me a rectal exam and that given my symptoms of discomfort, she probably should have administered a trans-vaginal ultrasound. I should have been more assertive and demanding as a patient, but today, I am focusing efforts on educating women and their medical care providers about ovarian cancer symptoms that appear "perimenopausal". These include pain during intercourse, digestive problems like bloating and nausea over an extended period of time, or soreness when touched that feels like a pulled muscle. I want them to remember my story, and that these symptoms could be signs of ovarian cancer.

WHILE PREGNANT

✦

Rachel

Diagnosed at age 40
In October 1994
With ovarian cancer
Stage IIIC

In 1993, I had been trying to get pregnant unsuccessfully for a year. That July, I had laparoscopic surgery to remove endometriomas on both my ovaries. I had taken Clomid for two cycles before getting pregnant, the following February.

During my sixth month of pregnancy, I told my doctors that I began experiencing excruciating pain in what felt like my ovaries. The doctors, however told me the pain was muscular, a symptom of pregnancy. Part of me doubted that I could really feel where my ovaries are, but deep down, I knew that the pain I was feeling was located there.

All my other symptoms could have been pregnancy-related as well: frequent urination, bloating, abdominal discomfort, nausea, gas, fatigue, backaches, and weight gain. In my 34th week of pregnancy, I went for a non-stress test, to check the baby's heart rate, because my doctor told me this was a routine procedure for 40 year old women like me. The test revealed that my baby's heart rate had plummeted. We were told we could watch it, but it kept happening. I stayed in the hospital, and they did an amniocentesis the next day to make sure my daughter's lungs were fully developed.

On an October evening, I received a C-section, as my doctor felt the baby was safer outside of my body than inside. After the procedure, she assured my husband and me that our baby girl was fine. We were allowed to hold our baby. The doctor continued the procedure and then told us that she thought there was something inside me that was not "deciduous to pregnancy."

I did not know what that meant. She called a pathologist and a gynecologic oncologist to the operating room. After they took a look and some biopsy samples, we were told that it was cancer. It was the best and the worst day of my life. My parents stood outside, worrying, and asked the pediatrician what was taking so long. She asked us what to say. We told her to tell them to wait.

The oncologist told us that he could not tell if the tumor had invaded my colon. He was certain, however, that it had spread throughout my abdominal cavity. I was put under general anesthesia and the gynecological oncologist performed an exploratory surgery. He was not able to remove the tumor, since he could not even reach the omentum with the C-section bikini type incision. He closed me up without removing anything. I was scheduled for a debulking surgery four days later, to remove the cancer.

The oncologist wanted me to move to the oncology floor, but I fought with him to let me stay with my baby until I had the surgery, on the maternity floor. He allowed me to stay.

During the debulking surgery, the gynecologic oncologist removed my ovaries, uterus, fallopian tube, appendix, and omentum. He told me it looked like borderline, not actually cancer, but the pathological report showed I had ovarian cancer stage IIIC.

After the surgery, I was moved to the oncology floor. Since I had come from the maternity ward, I had more flowers and cards than the oncology nurses had ever seen. I never felt more loved or supported in my life. I probably cried to every oncology nurse who worked there, during my treatment. My doctor told me I would see my daughter walk down the aisle one day. I asked him to reassure me of this many times, to help me get through my ordeal.

I went through six rounds of Taxol and Cisplatnin. Second look surgery revealed that one of 29 biopsies had microscopic evidence of cancer. I went through a second treatment of chemo, this time with a lower dose of intraperitoneal Taxol. I had third-look surgery, which revealed no traces of cancer. I thank God that I have been healthy ever since: 2004 was my tenth anniversary of being cancer-free. Despite my clean bill of health, I still have side effects from chemotherapy including gastrointestinal problems and neuropathy.

As a psychologist, I specialize in trauma recovery. I had never realized how traumatic going through such medical treatments could be for people. I have little memory of the two weeks following my C-section. It is only recently that I have been able to receive an injection without feeling the need to tell the clinician about my battle with cancer. I am fortunate that I had many cancer survivors in my family (mostly breast cancer but no ovarian cancer) who served as my role models. Throughout the whole experience, I always knew I was not going to let my daughter grow up without a mother. I always said that somebody had to be the one who survived this deadly disease. In addition, I realize now, with 10 years of hindsight, how much having cancer taught me about what is important in life.

DURABLE SURVIVOR'S
REAL HOPE

❖

Meg

Diagnosed at age 38
In 1995
With ovarian cancer
Stage IV

I had no symptoms of ovarian cancer, before my gynecologist detected a lump during a routine annual pelvic exam. She ushered me across the hall for an ultrasound that showed what she thought was simply "something on your ovary, probably just a dermoid cyst." Her calm was reinforced when my CA-125 came back normal. (My CA-125 has always been well within the normal range—as is true for about 20% of women diagnosed with ovarian cancer). What she thought was a cyst, was then burst during the laparoscopic surgery I underwent to remove it. A gynecologist—and not a gynecologic oncologist—performed the surgery since my HMO did not see the need to employ a gynecologic oncologist. They had informed that they would refer me to one if needed, and apparently, they did not feel it necessary. At that time, I didn't even know that gynecologic oncologists existed.

The pathologist's report said that while there was no cancer, there were cells of "low malignant potential" or "borderline" tumors. Later, I had these same slides reread for a second opinion. The second pathologist discovered not one, but *two* different ovarian cancer cell types in addition to the borderline tumor. At age 38, with children ages 1 and 3, and no history of cancer in my family, I was diagnosed with ovarian cancer. A couple of days later, I had a radical hysterectomy salpingo-oophorectomy (surgical removal of uterus, fallopian tubes, omentum, and ovaries) with a complete staging. While there were a couple of lesions on my uterus following this procedure, there were no more traces of cancer there or in the washings. I went home feeling sore, but relieved that I did not have to have chemo or radiation.

Three months later, I began to develop serious leg cramps and after a summer of taking pain medications and walking on crutches, my internist reluctantly agreed to order a Doppler scan of my legs and arms. Lo and behold, I had blood clots everywhere, including my lungs, and I was admitted to the hospital where, eventually, three lesions were discovered in my liver. Only one was biopsied, as they were precariously located near the dome of my liver—too close to my lungs and diaphragm for comfort. The news that the biopsy was positive (I have often thought it strange to call *that* "positive") for ovarian cancer came from my newly appointed oncologist who entered my room with a grim face and announced that things were "bad, very bad." I remember being completely baffled by his demeanor and, without thinking, grabbing him by the bow tie, and saying, "I don't think you understand me, I intend to live!" He extricated himself from my grasp and replied sarcastically, "Sure you do," and left. When the nurse came in a few minutes later, I told her I never wanted to see him again and she told me she would take care of it.

Before any surgery to remove the cancer in my liver could be considered, the blood clots issue had to be resolved. The course of action planned for me was to start chemo to reduce the tumor, which would hopefully also diminish the blood clots. My clotting was due to something called Trousseau's Syndrome, where certain types of cancer cause hyper coagulation, meaning excessive blood clotting. During surgery to install a chemo catheter in my chest, my left lung was accidentally punctured. When it became clear I could not breathe, an emergency procedure was performed in which a chest tube was stuck between my ribs, followed by my being hooked up to an inflating machine. Unfortunately, this all had to be repeated four days later when it was determined that the first chest tube was too small and a larger one was required. Finally, a week after what was supposed to be an outpatient procedure, I had my first round of chemo and went home.

Unfortunately, the "gold standard" chemotherapy was not effective against my tumors. After five cycles, the larger tumor had shrunk by only 10 percent and, since there was not much hope that chemo was going to improve the situation, I was scheduled for surgery to remove the tumors in my liver.

For some reason, I insisted on having a dye-injected scan called a portagram administered before my surgery. After reading the scan—and mercifully, before I had begun to drink the dreaded bowel prep cocktail—the liver surgeon entered my room with a grim face and told me that there were 12 visible lesions that existed in all three lobes of my liver. He explained that he could not do surgery under these circumstances, which would essentially turn my liver into Swiss cheese, making it certain that I would not survive. I remember his face; he was a young man, probably around my age, who had young children of his own. He clearly was sad and felt helpless; he even offered to talk with my children when, in the midst of tears, I asked what I could possibly tell them. Before he left my room, he said with authentic compassion, "Go home, and think about the quality, not the quantity, of your remaining days."

I did go home, but I did not think about the quality of my remaining days. I made appointments at five hospitals in three cities. My gynecologic oncologist had started me on a new regimen of oral chemotherapy. At first, I protested, thinking that surely, chemotherapy that could be administered orally could never work. But he assured me that he had some faith in this drug, so I took it. Besides, what other choice did I have?

My father and I formed an unusual team as we embarked together to visit five cancer centers in three cities, over the course of four days. In Los Angeles, we found a surgeon, a "buccaneer" by reputation. (But, as it was pointed out to us, we were in the market for a buccaneer.) He agreed to open me up and perform a procedure known as cryosurgery, meaning to freeze the tumors in my liver with liquid nitrogen. Even though he explained that the surgery would be very dangerous, we still made an appointment to return the following week to have it done. Before I arrived back home in Madison, WI, the surgeon had called to break the news that the Tumor Board at his hospital wouldn't allow him to operate on me unless I found a "smoking gun," a chemo that worked. I was angry and disappointed, but like the roller coaster that cancer treatment is, that did not last long. The next day I had my first CAT scan following the oral chemo, and the big tumor had shrunk by 50%! I called the Los Angeles doctor back and told him that we had his "smoking gun," and I was returned to the surgery schedule.

When I was finally on the operating table, an ultrasound of my liver revealed that there had only ever been one tumor in my liver. The other spots were cysts and blood density irregularities, common in about 10% of the population. The surgeon froze the tumor in my liver and closed me up. That was in March of 1995. Recently, my gynecologic oncologist dubbed me a "durable survivor."

A few months later, I began to think about what had happened to me. Had I gone home and thought about the "quality and not the quantity of my remaining days" I probably would have died, though later than expected, with loved ones remarking on what a testament that was to my will to live. No one would have known that I could have lived.

I attribute my survival to several things. First, I am an educated woman with a privileged upbringing who does not easily take "no" for an answer, particularly when it involves my own mortality. Second, I know that not even the most caring and intelligent professionals can know everything about a given problem. Therefore, the more intelligent individuals you have involved in your treatment, the better off you will be. I held the doors open when they appeared to be closing on me. Third, I attribute my survival to several physicians who were willing to risk their professional reputations and my life, and took chances that others would not. They were willing to have hope when hope was in short supply.

When I was diagnosed with cancer, it was as though I found myself in a boat in a tempest. The wind blew hard, and the waves sometimes were enormous. I would not survive alone, of course; there were many others in the boat with me: family, friends, physicians, nurses, and several oncologists. Often I was the captain I had the tiller, and could best steer the vessel. At other times, the best I could do was tremble down below, because the waves were too terrifying for me to watch. Many times, I felt someone else could better handle a particular wave, and I stepped aside and simply took an oar. For a patient with cancer, the ability to step aside and trust someone with your life is just as crucial as the ability to select carefully who that person will be.

We are not the ocean or the storm—neither patient nor physician can control the outcome. Although I have been cancer free for 10 years, I remain acutely aware that I may very well die of cancer at some point. I do not imagine that I have control of that monster. Still I do not have to give up control, because as it turns out, I never had it. Control is an illusion that we preserve to manage the randomness and chaos of life and death. What we must let go of then, is merely an illusion.

Patients with cancer do not need false hope, but neither do we need false and fatal abandonment of hope. We need to be brave enough to have real hope, and our physicians must have it as well. Real hope is born when patients and physicians let go of the illusion of control over the outcome without giving up. Real hope means staying invested in the outcome even though we know we cannot control it. Sometimes we are able to have an influence that changes the outcome, but that can happen only if we are willing to remain in the process while accepting the fact that we may die.

Each survivor has a story, an odyssey of survival. In addition, every one of those stories tells of people along the way, each one a link in the chain of survival. Almost daily, doctors have the opportunity to join someone's chain. But they cannot *be* the whole chain—they must not take on that impossible task. In the end, all of us can only do our best, and accept the fact that life is fragile and finite. Only after, we team up with our care providers, and give our best effort, can we rest assured there is nothing more we can do. Hindsight is always 20/20 and mistakes are a part of being human. In the end, what matters is that we do our best to honor the gift that is life.

CONCLUSIONS

◆

Ayala Miron

Ovarian cancer is highly curable when detected early. Women need to take action when they experience any unusual and persistent symptom, like the ones described in this book. They should trust their own body warning signs and seek thorough medical care immediately.

Most women with ovarian cancer do not have relatives with this disease. Ovarian cancer symptoms occur at the early stages of the disease. Even though the symptoms may not seem to be serious, they are the warning signs of ovarian cancer. Women, doctors, and nurses need to pay attention to them.

Ovarian Cancer Symptoms:

Changes in abdominal cramping, abnormal vaginal discomfort and bleeding, pain during sexual intercourse

- I began having periods that lasted 10 days and bad menstrual cramps. I had never suffered from bad menstrual cramps before, but the acute abdominal pains I started to feel, could literally stop me in my tracks.

- My menstrual cycles were lasting longer. I was getting mid-cycle spotting, vaginal aches, itching, and burning and repeated yeast infections. In the past, I had no trouble with my periods.

- I felt weird all the time, even worse around my period, weird pelvic cramping.

- Pelvic pain and spotting that I never had before.

- My period became irregular.

- I was having some discomfort during intercourse.

- The bleeding after the delivery of my child lasted longer than normal.

Abdominal or pelvic discomfort, unusual feeling of fullness, bloating, gas, nausea

- I had pain in my stomach and bowel.

- I began experiencing excruciating pain in what felt like my ovaries.

- I had experienced pelvic pain for about three months.

- I had a sharp pain attack in my lower right abdomen that lasted for a day it felt like a gallbladder attack.

- I felt queasy, had stomach, back, and pelvic pain, frequent urination, and bloating.

- I had pain in my stomach whenever I ate. My stomach pain became unbearable.

- I began having pains in my abdomen. These pains were like no other stomachache or cramp I had ever felt in my life.

- I felt pain in my lower left abdomen. I noticed it the most when I was doing sit-ups or when I was riding the exercise bicycle.

- I was feeling bloated and nauseous.

- The abdominal pain and bloating grew more acute.

- I was unable to eat more than a few mouthfuls. I complained that my stomach was upset, nothing major, but I was feeling a little achy. My lower abdomen continued to bother me.

- The pain had not subsided, and there was a lump in that same area of my abdomen where I was experiencing pain.

Indigestion, bowel changes, constipation, unexplained weigh loss, or gain

- My bowel movement habits gradually changed, they were getting thinner in size, and I had lost some weight.

- My lower abdominal pain was increasing a bit and my pants fit tighter.

- Although I was on a diet, my clothes were getting tight around the waist.

- I began gaining weight quickly, and it seemed like the weight was only going to my stomach area.

Increase in frequency of urination or urgency

- I felt "funny" and noticed that I felt pressure when I needed to urinate.
- I had the urge to urinate constantly.
- I had such urinary frequency, that I could not get a good night's sleep.

Shortness of breath, unusual fatigue

- I had a faint pain in my chest, repeatedly when taking deep breaths.
- The nausea started being accompanied by a shortness of breath, which occurred from time-to-time, but not consistently.
- Fatigued and a little bloated in the abdomen.
- I felt fatigue, bloated and that my stomach just did not feel right.

Unusual pain in hip, thighs, legs, lower backaches

- Weird pains in my thighs.
- I had aching, gnawing pains in my upper thighs and legs.
- I had frequent urination, hip pain, lower backaches, and shortness of breath.

Other symptoms

- I had nerve pain going through my right shoulder and down my arm that intensified when I took a deep breath.
- I felt as if I was getting the flu, only I would never come down with it, and then a week later I was getting something again.

Symptoms of ovarian cancer are often misdiagnosed as:

- Diverticulitis
- Irritable Bowel Syndrome (IBS)
- Gallbladder attack
- Sensitive bladder
- Perimenopause

- Ovarian cyst
- Emotional stress, depression

When one or more symptoms occur and persist, experts suggest to be followed closely with:

- Complete pelvic examination, including both bimanual pelvic exam and recto/vaginal exam
- CA-125 blood tests (unless a better test becomes available)
- Transvaginal ultrasounds

RESOURCES

OVARIAN CANCER RESOURCES

- **National Cancer Institute (NCI)**

  www.cancer.gov 1-800-4-CANCER (1-800-422-6237)

  Contains information about ovarian cancer and lists clinical trials open around the country. It also provides a list of comprehensive cancer centers in the US.

  To find the **NCI—Designated Comprehensive Cancer Centers List,** listed alphabetically by state, follow these steps:

  1. Log on the NCI website www.cancer.gov then.

  2. Enter the words, cancer center, in the search box and click on go.

  3. Under "Best bets for cancer centers" you will find "The National Cancer Institute Cancer Centers Program A fact sheet about National Cancer Institute-supported cancer centers" and click on it to get the full list.

  The NCI also provides up-to-date information over the phone on cancer care and clinical trials, 9am-4:30pm, Monday to Friday.

- **American Cancer Society (ACS)**

  www.cancer.org 1-800-ACS-2345 (1-800-227-2345)

  Provide free literature and help patients obtain financial and medical information.

  The ACS phone information service operates 24 hours 7 days a week.

- **PubMed**

  www.nlm.nih.gov.hinfo

  National library of medicine, database of medical journals.

- **American Society of Clinical Oncology**

  www.asco.org

  Information about ovarian cancer clinical trials research publications and referrals to gynecologic oncologists in your area.

- **Gynecologic Cancer Foundation**

  www.wcn.org

  Is a non-profit organization that is dedicated to educating women about ovarian cancer and other gynecologic cancers.

- **Medscape**

  www.medscape.com

  Information on ovarian cancer, registration is required but all information is free.

- **OncoLink**

  www.oncolink.upenn.edu

  This site offers information on ovarian cancer by the University of Pennsylvania.

PATIENT ADVOCACY ORGANISATIONS

- **Ovarian Cancer National Alliance (OCNA)**

  www.ovariancancer.org

  Working to increase public and professional understanding of ovarian cancer. It is also sponsoring the program—ovarian cancer survivors teaching medical students—were survivors give presentations, about ovarian cancer, to medical students, in medical schools nationwide.

  www.sandyovarian.org

  Ovarian cancer advocacy group also training ovarian cancer survivors for the presentations to medical students about ovarian cancer, in Philadelphia, PA.

- **National Ovarian Cancer Coalition (NOCC)**

  www.ovarian.org

Works to increase awareness of ovarian cancer and can connect newly diagnosed women with survivors in their area.

- **Ovarian Cancer Research Fund, Inc. (OCRF)**

www.ocrf.org

Funds research on early detection, diagnosis, and treatment of ovarian cancer.

- **SHARE**

www.sharecancersupport.org

Provides information hotline, peer-led support groups, wellness education, and advocacy programs.

- **The Center For Patient Partnerships**

University of Wisconsin-Madison

www.law.wisc.edu/patientadvocacy Phone: 608-265-6267

Provides information and services to help patients make decisions, in partnership with providers, and access the care they need and deserve. The Center advocates nationally for patient choices and preferences with health care providers, insurers, and other parties.

- **Gilda's Clubs**

www.gildasclub.org

Provides meeting places, lectures, workshops, and social events, to help build emotional and social support for ovarian cancer patients and their families and friends.

- **Association of Cancer Online Resources**

www.acor.org

Has a large ovarian cancer chat group, Ovarian Problem Discussion List, where patients often offer help and suggestions to other members.

- **The Wellness Community**

www.thewellnesscommunity.org

Facilities nationwide where one can find cancer support and education.

PUBLICATION FOR MEDICAL PROVIDERS ON OVARIAN CANCER SYMPTOMS

Frequency of Symptoms of Ovarian Cancer in Women Presenting to Primary Care Clinics. By Barbara A. Goff, MD, Lynn S. Mandel, PhD, Cindy H. Melancon, RN, Howard G. Muntz, MD. Published in JAMA, June 9, 2004, page 2705

PUBLICATIONS FOR PATIENTS AND CARE PROVIDERS

- **Ovarian Cancer—Your Guide to Taking Control** By Kristine Conner & Lauren Langford, Published by O'REILLY®, 2003

- **Conversations**

  www.ovarian-news.com

  A newsletter for those fighting ovarian cancer.

CANCER STATISTICS

❖

Source: American Cancer Society, 2004.

2004 ESTIMATED CANCER DEATHS OF WOMEN IN THE US

272,810 women are estimated to die of cancer in 2004.

25%   Lung & bronchus
15%   Breast
10%   Colon & rectum
 6%   Ovary
 6%   Pancreas
 4%   Leukemia
 3%   Non-Hodgkin lymphoma
 3%   Uterine corpus
 2%   Multiple myeloma
 2%   Brain/ONS
24%   All other sites

ONS=other nervous system.

2004 ESTIMATED CANCER CASES IN WOMEN IN THE US

668,470 women are estimated to be diagnosed with cancer in 2004.

32%   Breast
12%   Lung & bronchus
11%   Colon & rectum
 6%   Uterine corpus
 4%   Ovary
 4%   Non-Hodgkin lymphoma
 4%   Melanoma of skin
 3%   Thyroid
 2%   Pancreas
 2%   Urinary bladder
20%   All Other Sites

*Excludes basal and squamous cell skin cancers and in situ carcinomas except urinary bladder.

MEDICAL TERMS DICTIONARY

❖

Source: National Cancer Institute web site: www.cancer.gov

ascites (ah-SYE-teez)
Abnormal build-up of fluid in the abdomen that may cause swelling. In late-stage cancer, tumor cells may be found in the fluid in the abdomen. Ascites also occurs in patients with liver disease.

adenocarcinoma (AD-in-o-kar-sin-O-ma)
Cancer that begins in cells that line certain internal organs and that have glandular (secretory) properties.

barium enema
A procedure in which a liquid with barium in it is put into the rectum and colon by way of the anus. Barium is a silver-white metallic compound that helps to show the image of the lower gastrointestinal tract on an x-ray.

benign (beh-NINE)
Not cancerous. Benign tumors do not spread to tissues around them or to other parts of the body.

bladder
The organ that stores urine.

CA-125
A protein sometimes found in an increased amount in the blood that may suggest the presence of ovarian cancer.

cancer
A term for diseases in which abnormal cells divide without control. Cancer cells can invade nearby tissues and can spread through the bloodstream and lymphatic system to other parts of the body.

CAT scan
A series of detailed pictures of areas inside the body, taken from different angles; the pictures are created by a computer linked to an x-ray machine. Also called computerized axial tomography, computed tomography (CT scan), or computerized tomography.

CBC
Complete blood count. A test to check the number of red blood cells, white blood cells, and platelets in a sample of blood. Also called blood cell count.

chemotherapy (kee-mo-THER-a-pee)
Treatment with anticancer drugs.

clinical trial
A type of research study that uses volunteers to test new methods of screening, prevention, diagnosis, or treatment of a disease. The trial may be carried out in a clinic or other medical facility. Also called a clinical study.

cryosurgery (KRYE-o-SER-juh-ree)
Treatment performed with an instrument that freezes and destroys abnormal tissues.

cyst (sist)
A sac or capsule in the body. It may be filled with fluid or other material. Cysts are almost always benign

D&C
Dilation and curettage. A minor operation in which the cervix is expanded enough (dilation) to permit the cervical canal and uterine lining to be scraped with a spoon-shaped instrument called a curette (curettage). Also called dilatation and curettage.

debulking
Gynecologic oncologists use this as a verb to mean removal of tumor during surgery. For example: debulkig surgery, debulked, optimally debulked, suboptimally debulked etc…

diagnosis
The process of identifying a disease by the signs and symptoms.

diaphragm (DYE-a-fram)
The thin muscle below the lungs and heart that separates the chest from the abdomen

diverticulosis
A condition marked by small sacs or pouches (diverticula) in the walls of an organ such as the stomach or colon. These sacs can become inflamed and cause a

condition called diverticulitis, which may be a risk factor for certain types of cancer.

endometriosis (en-do-mee-tree-O-sis)
A benign condition in which tissue that looks like endometrial tissue grows in abnormal places in the abdomen

endometrium (en-do-MEE-tree-um)
The layer of tissue that lines the uterus

epithelial ovarian cancer (ep-ih-THEE-lee-ul)
Cancer that occurs in the cells lining the ovaries.

Epstein-Barr virus
EBV. A common virus that remains dormant in most people. It has been associated with certain cancers, including Burkitt's lymphoma, immunoblastic lymphoma, and nasopharyngeal carcinoma

fallopian tube (fa-LO-pee-in)
Part of the female reproductive tract. There are two long slender fallopian tubes through which eggs pass from the ovaries to the uterus.

fibroid (FYE-broyd)
A benign smooth-muscle tumor, usually in the uterus or gastrointestinal tract. Also called leiomyoma.

gene
The functional and physical unit of heredity passed from parent to offspring. Genes are pieces of DNA, and most genes contain the information for making a specific protein.

genetic
Inherited; having to do with information that is passed from parents to offspring through genes in sperm and egg cells.

high-dose chemotherapy
An intensive drug treatment to kill cancer cells, but that also destroys the bone marrow and can cause other severe side effects. High-dose chemotherapy is usually followed by bone marrow or stem cell transplantation to rebuild the bone marrow.

laparoscopy (lap-a-RAHS-ko-pee)
The insertion of a thin, lighted tube (called a laparoscope) through the abdominal wall to inspect the inside of the abdomen and remove tissue samples.

malignant (ma-LIG-nant)
Cancerous. Malignant tumors can invade and destroy nearby tissue and spread to other parts of the body.

mammogram (MAM-o-gram)
An x-ray of the breast.

medical oncologist (MED-i-kul on-KOL-o-jist)
A doctor who specializes in diagnosing and treating cancer using chemotherapy, hormonal therapy, and biological therapy. A medical oncologist often is the main health care provider for a person who has cancer. A medical oncologist also may coordinate treatment provided by other specialists.

MRI
Magnetic resonance imaging (mag-NET-ik REZ-o-nans IM-a-jing). A procedure in which radio waves and a powerful magnet linked to a computer are used to create detailed pictures of areas inside the body. These pictures can show the difference between normal and diseased tissue. MRI makes better images of organs and soft tissue than other scanning techniques, such as CT or x-ray. MRI is especially useful for imaging the brain, spine, the soft tissue of joints, and the inside of bones. Also called nuclear magnetic resonance imaging.

neuropathy
A problem in peripheral nerve function (any part of the nervous system except the brain and spinal cord) that causes pain, numbness, tingling, swelling, and muscle weakness in various parts of the body. Neuropathies may be caused by physical injury, infection, toxic substances, disease (e.g., cancer, diabetes, kidney failure, or malnutrition), or drugs such as anticancer drugs. Also called peripheral neuropathy.

omentum (oh-MEN-tum)
A fold of the peritoneum (the thin tissue that lines the abdomen) that surrounds the stomach and other organs in the abdomen

ovary (O-va-ree)
One of a pair of female reproductive glands in which the ova, or eggs, are formed. The ovaries are located in the pelvis, one on each side of the uterus.

pelvic exam
A physical examination of the vagina, cervix, uterus, fallopian tubes, ovaries, and rectum.

perimenopausal
The time of a woman's life when menstrual periods become irregular. Refers to the time near menopause.

peritoneum (PAIR-ih-toe-NEE-um)
The tissue that lines the abdominal wall and covers most of the organs in the abdomen.

port
An implanted device through which blood may be withdrawn and drugs may be infused without repeated needle sticks. Also called a port-a-cath.

remission
A decrease in or disappearance of signs and symptoms of cancer. In partial remission, some, but not all, signs and symptoms of cancer have disappeared. In complete remission, all signs and symptoms of cancer have disappeared, although cancer still may be in the body.

salpingo-oophorectomy (sal-PIN-go o-o-for-EK-toe-mee)
Surgical removal of the fallopian tubes and ovaries.

stage
The extent of a cancer within the body. If the cancer has spread, the stage describes how far it has spread from the original site to other parts of the body.

stage I ovarian cancer
Cancer is found in one or both of the ovaries and has not spread. Stage I is divided into stage IA, stage IB, and stage IC. In stage IA, cancer is found in a single ovary. In stage IB, cancer is found in both ovaries. In stage IC, cancer is found in one or both ovaries and one of the following is true: cancer is found on the outside surface of one or both ovaries; the capsule (outer covering) of the tumor has ruptured (broken open); or, cancer cells are found in fluid from the peritoneal cavity (the body cavity that contains most of the organs in the abdomen).

stage II ovarian cancer
Cancer is found in one or both ovaries and has spread into other areas of the pelvis. Stage II is divided into stage IIA, stage IIB, and stage IIC. In stage IIA, cancer has spread to the uterus and/or the fallopian tubes. In stage IIB, cancer has spread to other tissues within the pelvis. In stage IIC, cancer has spread to the uterus and/or fallopian tubes and/or other tissue within the pelvis and cancer cells are found in fluid from the peritoneal cavity (the body cavity that contains most of the organs in the abdomen).

stage III ovarian cancer
Cancer is found in one or both ovaries and has spread to other parts of the abdomen. Stage III is divided into stage IIIA, stage IIIB, and stage IIIC. In stage IIIA, the tumor is found in the pelvis only, but cancer cells have spread to the surface of the peritoneum. In stage IIIB, cancer has spread to the peritoneum but is not larger than 2 centimeters in diameter. In stage IIIC, cancer has spread to the peritoneum and is larger than 2 centimeters in diameter and/or has spread to lymph nodes in the abdomen. Cancer that has spread to the surface of the liver is also considered stage III disease.

stage IV ovarian cancer
Cancer is found in one or both ovaries and has metastasized (spread) beyond the abdomen to other parts of the body. Cancer that is found in tissues of the liver is considered stage IV disease.

stem cell
A cell from which other types of cells can develop.

stem cell transplantation
A method of replacing immature blood-forming cells that were destroyed by cancer treatment. The stem cells are given to the person after treatment to help the bone marrow recover and continue producing healthy blood cells.

symptom
An indication that a person has a condition or disease. Some examples of symptoms are headache, fever, fatigue, nausea, vomiting, and pain.

transvaginal ultrasound
A procedure used to examine the vagina, uterus, fallopian tubes, ovaries, and bladder. An instrument is inserted into the vagina, and sound waves bounce off organs inside the pelvic area. These sound waves create echoes, which a computer uses to create a picture called a sonogram. Also called TVS.

thrombocyte (THROM-bo-site)
A blood cell that helps prevent bleeding by causing blood clots to form. Also called a platelet.

ultrasound
A procedure in which high-energy sound waves (ultrasound) are bounced off internal tissues or organs and make echoes. The echo patterns are shown on the screen of an ultrasound machine, forming a picture of body tissues called a sonogram. Also called ultrasonography.

uterus (YOO-ter-us)
The small, hollow, pear-shaped organ in a woman's pelvis. This is the organ in which a fetus develops. Also called the womb.

ABOUT THE AUTHOR

Ayala Miron was born and raised in Israel. As a child, she also lived in France and spent time visiting her family in the US. After high school, she was drafted and served in the Israeli Air Force as a paramedic sergeant. Ms. Miron earned a B.S. in Civil Engineering from the Technion, Israel Institute of Technology, in Haifa. There she met her husband Ami and together they moved to the United States and started their family. Ayala earned a Masters degree in Computer Science from Pace University New York, New York.

Ayala worked as Civil engineer in New York State and earned her P.E. (Professional Engineer) license there. When her second son was born, she stopped working to be with her children. She dedicates most of her time to raising and caring for her four children: Benjamin, Jonathan, Michelle, and David. She lives with her family in a suburb of Philadelphia, Pennsylvania.

The author can be reached by email at:
ayala@ocjourneys.com

0-595-33031-2

Printed in the United States
100018LV00005B/344/A